Federal Pharmacy Law
2nd Edition

Barry S. Reiss, Ph.D.
Professor Emeritus
Albany College of Pharmacy
Albany, New York

Gary D. Hall, M.S.
Professor of Pharmaceutics
Albany College of Pharmacy
Albany, New York

Apothecary Press
Delmar, New York
2001

Notice: The authors of this volume have prepared this publication to provide accurate and authoritative information about federal pharmacy law as of the date of publication. The authors and publisher disclaim all responsibility for any liability, loss, injury, or damage incurred as a consequence, directly or indirectly, of the use and application of any of the contents of this volume. The reader is advised to review original law sources if in doubt about any statement made in this work.

 For information, address Apothecary Press, 10 Parkwyn Circle, Delmar, New York, 12054-4135
www.apothecarypress.com

Library of Congress Card Number: 2001086671

ISBN 0-9676332-1-4

Printed in the United States of America

Table of Contents

Preface

On behalf of Apothecary Press and the authors, we welcome you to our Guide to Federal Pharmacy Law, 2nd Edition. This Guide has been prepared to assist you in making the review of federal law as simple and painless as possible.

The Guide is divided into fourteen sections, each of which is designated with a letter. Within some sections there are sample questions similar to the type that may be seen on the MPJE®. Answers to these questions are provided immediately below the questions.

At the end of this Guide are 250 multiple-choice questions that cover the federal statutes addressed by this book. Candidates are encouraged to attempt to answer these questions only after they have completed studying the contents of this Guide. This will serve as a practice examination that will help to identify areas of weakness that require further study. Answers to these questions may be found at the very end of the question section.

At the end of this Guide is a list of names, addresses, and phone numbers of the State Boards of Pharmacy in the United States. Candidates are advised to first contact the board of pharmacy in the state(s) in which they plan to seek licensure in order to obtain the latest information about specific state requirements.

Barry S. Reiss
Gary D. Hall

Section A

Guide to the MPJE®

Applying for and Taking the MPJE®

The MPJE® is a computerized law examination, which must be taken in order to obtain a pharmacist license in most states. The examination consists of questions based upon the Federal Drug Law Examination (FDLE) and each individual state's laws and regulations.

All candidates are advised to obtain the latest copy of the MPJE® Registration Bulletin available from the

National Association of Boards of Pharmacy
700 Busse Highway
Park Ridge, Illinois 60068
Telephone (847) 698-6227
www.nabp.net

This bulletin is updated on a regular basis and describes the procedures for applying for and taking the computerized examination. You may also wish to purchase their Candidate's Review Guide. Request ordering information and pricing from NABP's Publications Desk at the above telephone number.

Remember that each individual state has established its own criteria for determining a candidate's eligibility to take the law examination. However, the following guidelines may simplify your application process:

- Carefully review the NABP's Registration Bulletin because changes may be made to the guidelines at any time.

- Complete the registration form and mail it to your STATE BOARD OF PHARMACY with the required fees. Be sure to apply for the appropriate examination (i.e. either the NAPLEX® or the MPJE®)

- Your state's board of pharmacy will notify NABP of your eligibility to take the examination.

- If you are qualified to take an examination, an Authorization to Test (ATT) will be sent to you. It will indicate the dates of your eligibility, an ATT number, a candidate identification number, and an expiration date (usually about 1 year).

- You may contact any testing center location to schedule your individual testing time. Presently Sylvan Technology Centers are being used. When contacting the testing site, have the following available:

    - authorization number
    - candidate ID number
    - expiration date from your ATT card

- Arrive at the testing center at least 15 minutes early. Have available:

    - your ATT

- two forms of identification, at least one of which must have a picture ID with signature. (Driver's license or passport acceptable)

- The computerized examination must be completed in two hours. Extra time will be provided to complete a questionnaire and a short tutorial.

- No food, drink, reference books, or notes are allowed. You are not permitted to open personal belongings such as purses or wallets during the exam.

- Your examination score will be reported only to your state's Board of pharmacy.

Content of the MPJE®

The MPJE® examination will most likely consist of 90 multiple-choice questions of which 60 will contribute to your score. The remaining 30 are intermingled throughout the exam and are "pretest questions". That is, they are new questions, which the NABP is evaluating for level of difficulty and appropriateness. Some of these may show up in later examinations as questions that will count!

The level of difficulty for MPJE® questions will vary. While the passing score for the exam is set at 75, it does NOT mean that you have to correctly answer at least 75% of the questions in order to pass. The actual number of correct answers needed to pass a specific examination will vary from one exam to another. The person next to you may have some questions that are different from yours in wording, topics covered, and degree of difficulty. The cardinal rule to remember is simply to answer ALL questions to the best of your ability. Do not become discouraged if you have several very difficult questions.

The examination will have questions involving federal laws and regulations as well as specific state laws and regulations. The questions will be intermingled. Clearly, you should be familiar with not only the federal laws and regulations, but also those of the state to which you are applying. Because each state has its own unique laws, this Guide is focused only on federal laws and regulations.

MPJE® Competency Statements

The NABP has established the following competency statements for their federal drug examination:

Area 1 Pharmacy Practice
(approximately 78 % of the exam)

1.01 Identify the legal responsibilities of the pharmacist and other pharmacy personnel.

1.02 Identify requirements for acquisition and distribution of pharmaceutical products.

1.03 Identify legal requirements that must be observed in the issuance of a prescription or a drug order.

1.04 Identify the procedures necessary to properly dispense a pharmaceutical product including controlled substances.

1.05 Identify the conditions for making an offer to counsel or counseling appropriate patients.

1.06 Identify requirements for distribution or dispensing of nonprescription products, including controlled substances.

1.07 Identify the proper procedures for keeping records of information related to pharmaceutical products including requirements for protecting patient confidentiality.

Area 2 Licensure, Registration, Certification, and Operational Requirements
(approximately 17 % of the exam)

2.01 Identify the qualifications, application procedure, necessary examinations, and internship requirements for licensure, registration, or certification of individuals engaged in the manufacture, storage, distribution, and/or dispensing of pharmaceutical products.

2.02 Identify the requirements and application procedure for the registration, licensure, certification, or permitting of a practice setting or business entity.

2.03 Identify the operational requirements for the registration, licensure, certification, or permitting of a practice setting (e.g., space, equipment, advertising and signage, automated equipment, storage, and security).

Area 3 Regulatory Structure and Terms
(approximately 5% of exam)

3.01 Identify the purpose of and the terms and conditions found in the laws and rules that regulate or affect the manufacture, storage, distribution, and dispensing of pharmaceutical products.

3.02 Identify the authority, responsibilities, and operation of the agencies or entities that enforce the laws and rules.

Study Tip

After reading the above carefully constructed objectives, what have you learned? Probably not a great deal, since most of the objectives are very general and do not focus on specific items. That is all right. Hopefully we will review material most likely to be on your exam. Naturally there will always be a few questions from "left field" that were neither presented in this Guide or in your pharmacy college's jurisprudence course. Don't worry about the isolated facts. Instead concentrate on major topics. Also remember that this Guide reviews only federal law. Approximately 50% of your exam will be based upon state law. You are fortunate if you are taking the exam in a state that follows federal law closely.

Study Tip

In reviewing for the exam, your objective is to learn the law and to recognize what areas of the law are applicable in a particular question. DO NOT attempt to memorize the exact citation for a law such as 503; 21 U.S.C. 353 for the Durham-Humphrey Amendment or a state regulation designation such as "Section 2857" of the Public health law. While it may be useful to learn the date of origin for major laws such as the FD&C Act of 1938, it is very unlikely that you will be specifically questioned on the dates of less significant legislation.

Remember also that when legislation is passed it may not immediately take effect. For example the Durham-Humphrey Amendment was passed by Congress in 1951 but did not become effective until 1952. Spend the majority of your review time on questions related to the federal Controlled Substances Act. Obviously it is also important to concentrate on your individual state's pharmacy laws.

Tips For Answering Test Questions

Questions on the MPJE® are likely to be in one of two formats. Many questions will have a simple stem followed by five choices lettered A through E. the candidate must select the BEST answer and key that answer into the computer. Other questions will be multi-response questions or "K" questions. This refers to questions with a simple stem followed by three choices numbered I, II, and III. The answer choices will consist of several single and combinations of these three choices. The format always used for answer choices in "K" questions is:

(A) I only (B) III only (C) I and II only
(D) II and III only (E) I, II, and III

"K" questions are frequently found on the NAPLEX® and to a lesser degree on the MPJE®. These questions are usually considered to be more difficult than standard multiple-choice questions since the candidate is not just seeking a single correct answer but possible combinations of correct answers. While many federal laws and regulations are complex, MPJE® examiners are generally realistic and are unlikely to ask the candidate to identify obscure facts about federal laws.

Study Tip

When answering a "K" question, ignore the combinations of answers until you have closely evaluated each choice. For each, decide if it is true or correct, and then hope that your answer is in the key. For example, if you decide that I and II are correct answers and III is not, obviously you would key in (C) as the answer. However if you have selected the combination of I and III, you will quickly notice that this combination is not in the answer key. Obviously you should reconsider as to whether just I or III are correct or if it is possible that II is also correct? A second situation occurs when you have decided that III is correct, I is not correct, but you are uncertain about choice II. It is probably better to go with what you know to be correct, i.e., the choice of III only.

Other things to remember while you are taking the MPJE® include:

- Read each question carefully and try to determine what concept, general principle or specific law is being tested. Remember that when there is a conflict between federal and an individual state's law, the stricter usually applies (e.g. if a controlled drug is federally classified in Schedule III and is classified by the state as a Schedule II drug, the more stringent state law applies)

- When a question mentions a specific drug, try to classify it in your mind as a controlled substance, non-controlled prescription-only drug or OTC.

- Assume that each question is written in a straightforward manner. The examiners are not out to trick you.

- After deciding upon the correct response, complete the answering process using three steps.

  - Highlight the answer on the computer screen.

  - Request the next question by keying the icon on the lower right portion of the screen.

  - Confirm that you want the next question by keying the icon next to the above icon.

Note

Remember that once you have completed steps 2 and 3, you are not permitted to return to the previous question and change your answer. Don't hurry through questions and risk a quick decision. You have plenty of time to complete the examination. On the other hand, don't overanalyze the questions. Your first choice is probably the best choice

Scoring of your MPJE® is done very quickly and the results are sent to the board(s) of pharmacy you have designated. Remember that you have no way of knowing how well you are doing during the exam. Do not become discouraged if you run into several difficult questions. Simply answer ALL questions to the best of your ability and knowledge. While the passing grade is set at 75%, this does not mean that you have to correctly answer a minimum of 75% of the questions. It is possible that a raw score of below 75% will convert into a passing grade.

Common Errors Made By Candidates

- ***Not reading the question carefully***

  Example: Which one of the following is NOT required to be placed by the pharmacist onto a prescription?

  vs.

  Which one of the following is NOT required to be placed by the pharmacist onto a prescription label?

- ***Applying local laws or regulations***

  Example: Expiration dating on prescription labels is NOT required by either federal or most state laws but may be a local requirement.

- ***Basing your answers on what you do in the pharmacy you are employed in***

  Unfortunately, many pharmacies do not follow the letter of the law. Using daily practice as a guideline for your answer may result in wrong answers on this examination.

- ***Attempting to base an answer on recent changes in the law.***

  New laws or regulations may be ambiguous or poorly understood by practitioners. For this reason questions on the MPJE® exam are usually based on well established laws and regulations. If a question is based on a fairly recent law it is likely to be a question that is being tested by NABP and will likely not count toward your score.

Section B

Sources of Laws, Rules and Regulations

Introduction

Many laws and amendments that have shaped the current Food, Drug and Cosmetic Act were enacted over the past 100 years. In most cases they represent attempts on the part of lawmakers to protect the American public.

Pure Food and Drug Act of 1906

Up to 1906 there were relatively few controls on the distribution of foods, drug-containing products, cosmetic products and medical devices. Products were often contaminated, were not consistent in strength and were poorly labeled. In 1906 Congress passed the Pure Food and Drug Act. This law prohibited foods and drugs that were distributed through interstate commerce to be adulterated or misbranded. The law fell short of protecting the public since it did not require manufacturers to list ingredients or directions for use of a product on the label. The law also did not regulate cosmetic products or medical devices.

Food, Drug and Cosmetic Act of 1938

In 1937, 107 deaths caused by the mistaken use, by the manufacturer of diethylene glycol (automobile antifreeze), as a vehicle in a sulfanilamide elixir resulted in the passage of a landmark piece of federal regulation, the Food, Drug and Cosmetic Act (FDCA) of 1938. The law required, for the first time in the US, that any new drug could not be marketed unless it had first been proven to be safe when used according to directions on the label. It also required that labels include adequate directions for use and warnings about habit-forming drugs that were contained in the product. It was also the first law that applied to cosmetic products and medical devices as well as to food and drug products. Drug products marketed prior to 1938 were exempted or "grandfathered" from the law and did not, therefore, have to be labeled or proven safe under this law. The FDCA became the backbone of many subsequent laws and amendments that further strengthened drug control in the US.

Note

Several drug products still sold in pharmacies (e.g. levothyroxine, digoxin, nitroglycerin, and phenobarbital) were on the market prior to 1938 and are therefore still "grandfathered" from this law.

Durham-Humphrey Amendment of 1951

Many of the drug products covered by the 1938 FDCA Act were not safe to use without medical supervision. The Durham-Humphrey Amendment of 1951 was enacted to further regulate these products. This was an amendment to the FDCA that established two classes of drugs. Those that required medical supervision to be used safely did not have to list "adequate directions for use" but were required to include the legend "Caution: Federal law prohibits dispensing without a prescription" on the manufacturer's label.

The requirement for "adequate directions for use" was satisfied by the pharmacist placing on the label of the dispensed product, directions provided by the prescriber (e.g. Take one tablet twice daily). Such products became known as prescription or "legend" drugs. Products that did not require medical supervision for their use had to have adequate directions for use on their label and were referred to as "over-the-counter" or nonprescription drug products. In addition to distinguishing between legend and nonprescription drug products, this legislation also provided for oral prescriptions and prescription refills.

Kefauver-Harris Amendment of 1962

The Kefauver-Harris Amendment was adopted as a result of public concern about thalidomide, a tranquilizer drug marketed primarily in Europe. This drug was marketed in Europe but was not approved by the FDA for the US market. In 1961, it was determined that thalidomide had caused serious birth defects in the offspring of many women in Europe who had used the drug.

While there were few birth defects seen in the US, Congress enacted the Kefauver-Harris Amendment to protect the public in the future. This amendment to the FDCA Act (also referred to as the Drug Efficacy Amendment) required that all new drugs marketed in the US had to be shown to be not only safe but also effective. This requirement was also extended to products that had been approved between 1938 and 1962.

In addition to this efficacy requirement, the amendment also included provisions that placed the authority for regulating prescription drug advertising into the hands of the FDA. It also required informed consent for individuals who were research subjects in clinical investigations, reporting of adverse drug reactions, and creation of Good Manufacturing Practices (GMP) requirements that clearly defined the conditions under which drugs could be manufactured in the US.

Medical Device Amendment of 1976

In order to protect the American public against potentially dangerous or useless medical devices, Congress enacted the Medical Device Amendment of 1976. This amendment to the FDCA Act provides for better classification of medical devices according to their specific function, establishment of performance standards for these devices, pre-market approval requirements, conformance with GMP standards, and requirements for adherence to record and reporting requirements.

Orphan Drug Act of 1983

Orphan drugs are those that are used to treat diseases that affect relatively few people. Prior to 1983 the cost of developing and marketing such drugs was prohibitive for most drug manufacturers because of their limited potential for profitability. In 1983 Congress enacted the Orphan Drug Act. This provided various tax and licensing incentives to manufacturers that made development of such drugs more appealing.

Drug Price Competition and Patent-Term Restoration Act of 1984

This piece of legislation, sometimes called the Waxman-Hatch Amendment, attempted to resolve a dispute between generic drug and brand name drug manufacturers. Prior to the enactment of this amendment to the FDCA, generic drug manufacturers had to go through most of the lengthy drug approval process that was required of manufacturers of newly developed drugs. New drug manufacturers were concerned about limited periods of exclusive patent rights for their innovative products. In enacting this bill, Congress streamlined the drug approval process for generic drugs and provided innovative drug manufacturers with incentives to develop new drug products.

Prescription Drug Marketing Act of 1987

This bill was enacted in order to place more stringent controls on the distribution of prescription drugs samples and to prevent hospitals and other health care entities from reselling pharmaceuticals to other businesses. It was an attempt to more precisely manage the drug distribution system in the US.

FDA Modernization Act of 1997

This Act is a far-reaching piece of legislation that touches virtually every aspect of FDA's activities. Included in this legislation are:

- Provisions for the fast-track review of some New Drug Application submissions. The intent is to expedite the approval of new drugs used to treat serious or life-threatening conditions.

- Clarification of the conditions under which pharmacies may perform extemporaneous compounding of prescriptions. One premise is that individual states should regulate compounding. Also pharmacies are exempt from the strict regulatory federal GMP standards and the requirements for submission of new drug applications.

- The prescription drug legend "Caution: Federal law prohibits dispensing without a prescription" is replaced by "Rx only".

- The provision that required certain substances to be labeled "Warning – May be habit forming." has been eliminated.

- Encouragement for manufacturers to conduct research for new uses of drugs and to submit supplemental NDA's for these uses. The manufacturers may publicly disseminate limited information on these unapproved uses provided a statement is included specifying that the use has not been approved or cleared by the FDA.

Official Compendia

- **United States Pharmacopoeia/National Formulary (USP/NF)**

The US government does NOT publish this reference. It is published by a private organization known as the US Pharmacopoeia Convention (USPC). The USP/NF contains monographs of recognized drugs that include their chemical characteristics and standards of quality. Proposed changes in revisions of the USP/NF are published in The Pharmacopeial Forum (PF), a bimonthly publication.

- **Homeopathic Pharmacopoeia of the United States (HPUS)**

  This is also published by a private organization or convention that updates information concerning homeopathic products or remedies on a regular basis.

Note

If a drug is listed by its official name in the USP/NF or HPUS, it must meet the requirements specified in either book. Otherwise, it must have the designation "not USP/NF". Without this designation the drug is considered to be either misbranded or adulterated.

Pure Food + Drug 1906
↳ unadulterated products

Food Drug + Cosmetic 1938
(Safe drugs (Grandfather clause)

Durham Humphrey 1951
Difference b/w OTC/Rx
"Legend" developed
Oral Rx's

Kefaver-Harris 1962
- Safe + Effective

FDA Modernization 1997
- Fast track approval
- Rx only
- Encourages SNDA's

Section C

Acronyms and Definitions

The pharmacist is expected to have a working knowledge of health care terminology. It is, therefore, frustrating when one encounters an unfamiliar abbreviation or acronym. Throughout this Guide, we will use such abbreviations or acronyms. The following table will be a useful guide to those most popularly used:

Study Tip

Fortunately, the MPJE® is a multiple-choice exam so that you will not likely be asked to give the name of the organization with the acronym "HCFA". However, a question could be worded: "What federal organization is responsible for administering Medicare?" Another question might be "Which Federal department is responsible for the DEA?" (The Department of Justice). It is probably sufficient if you review the following list and simply be able to recognize the meaning of these common acronyms. It is unlikely that any deliberate "trick" question will be asked, such as "Is HCFA an administration or an agency?"

Acronyms

AAC	Actual Acquisition Cost - the actual price a pharmacist pays when purchasing units of a drug product. This price usually represents a discounted price from the average wholesale price (AWP).
ADE or ADR	Adverse drug experience or adverse drug reaction
ATF	Alcohol, Tobacco, and Firearms agency
AWP	Average wholesale price – a published wholesale price for a drug that can be used as the basis for pricing prescription drugs. Usually pharmacies are able to purchase the drug at lower (discounted) prices from the AWP.
CDC	Centers for Disease Control
CFR	Code of Federal Regulations - a compilation of final regulations and notices promulgated by the federal government; published annually by the Government Printing Office; the above regulations and notices are first published in the Federal Register, a daily publication.
CPSC	Consumer Product Safety Commission
DEA	Drug Enforcement Administration - administration responsible for the Federal Controlled Substances Act; part of the U.S. Department of Justice

DHHS	Department of Health and Human Services - department which includes the FDA
DME	Durable Medical Equipment – equipment that meets three standards: 1. It can stand repeated use 2. It is primarily for a medical purpose (i.e., it is not useful to a person if they have no illness or injury) 3. It is appropriate for use in the home Examples include wheelchairs, oxygen tanks
DRG's	Diagnosis Related Groups - a classification system for hospital inpatients based on the principle diagnosis; reimbursement is usually based on days of stay.
DUR	Drug Utilization Review – a review of prescription drug use, prescriber prescribing patterns or drug utilization by patients. Purpose is to determine if appropriate drugs are being prescribed and if those drugs are being used appropriately.
EAC	Estimated acquisition cost – an estimated cost of a drug based upon information collected by the DHHS (Dept. of Health and Human Services). Many costs are based upon volume of drug sales.
FDA	Food and Drug Administration

FDCA	Food, Drug, and Cosmetic Act (FD & C Act, FDCA)
FTC	Federal Trade Commission - responsible for investigating unfair business practices including misleading advertising, etc.
GMP	Good manufacturing practices
GRAS	Generally recognized as safe - refers to a large number of relatively inert ingredients that are permitted to be used in pharmaceutical and food products as excipients or adjuvants because of their relatively high degree of safety
GRASE	Generally recognized as safe and effective - term usually used when considering nonprescription products
HCFA	Health Care Financing Administration - responsible for policies relating to Medicare (federally managed) and Medicaid (controlled by individual states under the supervision of HCFA)
HHA	Home Health Agency – an organization licensed or certified by the government to provide home health care
HMO	Health maintenance organization
HP or HPUS	Homeopathic Pharmacopoeia of the

	United States
JCAHO	Joint Commission on Accreditation of Health Care Organizations
MAC	Maximum allowable cost – the highest price allowed under a specific plan for a specific drug (usually multi-source drugs). If a person wants a more expensive version, he must pay the difference.
NAPB	National Association of Boards of Pharmacy - responsible for the preparation of both the NAPLEX® and MPJE®
NDC	National drug code – a classification system for identifying a specific drug product; used nationally for reimbursement and for identification of drug products.
NIH	National Institutes of Health
OBRA	Omnibus Budget Reconciliation Act - acts passed each year by Congress for funding many activities, each OBRA known by the year it is enacted.
OSHA	Occupational Safety and Health Administration - monitors work environment to assure worker safety.
OTC	Over-the-Counter - refers to drugs and

	drug products, which are available without a prescription
PBM	Pharmacy Benefits Manager
PHS	Public Health Service
PI	Package insert
PPI	Patient package insert
PPO	Preferred Provider Organization – a group of health professionals who by contract are favored in providing health services to individuals under a specific insurance plan.
PPPA	Poison Prevention Packaging Act
SDA	Specially denatured alcohol
SNF	Skilled Nursing Facility - a site that treats patients especially in need of rehabilitation or a lower level of medical care than that needed in a hospital.
TRP	Tamper resistant packaging
USAN	United States Adopted Names
USP/NF	*United States Pharmacopoeia/ National Formulary*

USP DI

U*nited States Pharmacopoeia Dispensing Information* - a set of three volumes containing a variety of information. They include

Volume I - Drug Information for the Health Care Professional - contains information about individual drugs written for health professionals.

Volume II - Advice for the Patient - Drug information in lay language - contains information intended for the general public about the use of drugs, side effects, etc; individual pages may be photocopied and given to patients as part of a counseling process

Volume III - Approved Drug Products With Therapeutic Equivalence Evaluations - contains information from the Orange Book, USP regulations, portions of the Federal Controlled Substances Act, plus other information.

Definitions

Cosmetic

Article intended to be rubbed, poured, sprinkled, sprayed on, introduced into or otherwise applied to the human body for the purpose of cleansing, beautifying, promoting attractiveness, or altering the appearance. Also, any component of the above articles is considered to be a cosmetic.

> **Note**
>
> There is one exception to the above - soap is not considered to be a cosmetic.

Device

Any instrument, apparatus, implement, machine, contrivance, implant, *in vitro* reagent or related article which is

- recognized in the USP/NF or HP or any supplement

- intended for use in the diagnosis, cure, mitigation, treatment, or prevention of disease in man or other animals

- intended to affect the structure or any function of the body of humans or animals but are not foods

Note

Examples of devices would include infusion pumps, cardiac pacemakers, heart monitors, etc.

Drug

1. Article recognized in the official United States Pharmacopoeia (USP/NF) official National Formulary (NF), or official Homeopathic Pharmacopoeia of the United States (HPUS), or any supplements of these references
2. Article intended for use in the diagnosis, cure, mitigation, treatment, or prevention of disease in man or other animals
3. Article (other than food) intended to affect the structure or any function of the body of man or other animals
4. Article intended for use as a component of any articles specified in the above but does not include devices or their components, parts, or accessories.

Food

An article used for food or drink in humans or animals, chewing gum, and substances used as components of food or drink.

Note

It is unlikely that questions concerning subtle distinctions between foods, drugs, and cosmetics will be asked since there have been too many court decisions and changing opinions. For example, minor claims for "anti-aging" creams have been accepted for cosmetic status while other creams containing hormones are considered to be drug products. Also, some chemicals with therapeutic uses have been classified as dietary supplements.

Generic name A name that is assigned to a specific drug structure. It is a simplified name as compared to the chemical name. Drug products may be marketed under the "generic name" or a brand name (trade name). Overall implication is that a drug marketed under the generic name only is less expensive than the brand name product.

Hospice A facility or program that provides palliative and supportive care for terminally ill patients.

Section D

Bringing New Drugs to Market

Investigational New Drug Application (IND)

Before a new drug is marketed a sponsor (usually a manufacturer) has to complete an extensive testing process to assure that the new drug will be safe and effective for what it is claimed to do. The Investigational New Drug Application (IND) is the first application form that a sponsor must submit to the FDA before a drug may be administered to humans. The requirement for an IND approval is intended to protect both the rights and safety of humans upon whom the drug will be tested.

While most sponsors are pharmaceutical companies, it is possible for a medical researcher, academic personnel, or organizations, either public or private, to submit INDs. Once submitted, the FDA has 30 days in which to decide whether the investigational drug is suitable for testing.

Virtually all of the information collected by the sponsor, especially from preclinical (animal) studies, which reflect on both the use and safety of the proposed investigational drug, is submitted to the FDA as part of the IND application. In addition, the sponsor must provide complete descriptions of the methodology (clinical protocols) to be used in testing the drugs in humans.

Clinical Trials

After the FDA approves an IND, the sponsor may initiate clinical (human) trials. There are three phases before the final approval of the drug and one additional phase after the drug product has been marketed. The drug must satisfactorily complete each phase before it can progress to the next.

- Phase 1 A small group of healthy individuals is given the drug. The primary purpose of this phase is to evaluate the drug's toxicological, pharmacokinetic and pharmacological properties, as well as to assess the safety of the drug in humans.

- Phase 2: A larger group (100 or more) of patients that have the disease or symptoms of the condition claimed to be treated by the drug is given the new drug. The purpose of this phase is to determine the effectiveness of the drug and to obtain information about adequate dosage, relative safety, and adverse effects.

- Phase 3: Large groups of patients (sometimes thousands) in several geographical locations are part of controlled clinical studies. The purpose of this phase is to obtain data concerning the drug's effectiveness as compared to a control group that receives a placebo. Most Phase 3 studies are double-blinded (i.e. neither the patient or investigator knows whether the drug or placebo is being given until after the study is completed)

Phase 1 and 2 studies are usually conducted under the direct supervision of the sponsoring company while Phase 3 studies usually involve testing performed at remote and varied clinical sites by independent investigators. Obviously Phase 3 studies are the most costly and take an extended period of time to complete. In each of these first three phases the patient or their representative must provide informed consent, i.e. they must agree to be subjects in the testing program after having been advised of the potential risks.

Treatment Investigational New Drugs

Treatment INDs allow the administration of an investigational new drug to patients that have not been enrolled in the new drug's clinical trials program. These patients must be in an imminent life-threatening stage of an illness for which there is presently no cure or where the presently used drugs do not appear to be effective. Examples of such diseases might be advanced stages of AIDS, some cancers, Alzheimer's disease, and Parkinson's disease.

The company developing the drug must have presented data outlining the drug's safety and efficacy, and the drug must be in either Phase 2 or 3 of clinical trials. If the drug is being considered as a Treatment IND candidate, a "treatment protocol" must be submitted to the FDA, which describes its proposed use in the designated patients.

The New Drug Application (NDA) Process

Once sufficient data concerning drug efficacy, toxicity, stability, production methods, packaging and the data from numerous clinical trials on patients have been collected, a new drug application may be submitted to the FDA for review. If the FDA reviewers are satisfied with the accuracy and completeness of the data from the clinical trials (Phases 1, 2 and 3), the NDA is approved and the NDA will be "on file" at the FDA. At this point the manufacturer may market the new drug product.

The NDA often consists of thousands of pages of data and information and is very costly and time-consuming to prepare. Once submitted, the FDA generally reviews the application for at least six months and provides experts and other interested parties the opportunity to comment on the submission.

After the drug product is marketed, Phase 4 studies are conducted. This is the post-marketing surveillance of the drug. During this period, health professionals are encouraged to report any problems with the drug, especially adverse effects experienced when the drug is used. The drug manufacturer must also submit yearly reports concerning new information and field reports concerning the drug product. The FDA utilizes Phase 4 data to determine whether or not a product should remain on the market.

Abbreviated New Drug Application (ANDA)

Before any new drug may be placed on the market, the innovator company must submit the data described for IND's and NDA's. Usually the innovator pharmaceutical company will have patent protection for their drug entity. However, once the patent expires, other companies may wish to introduce the drug under the drug's generic name only or as a brand name product. Rather than requiring the secondary companies to submit a complete NDA, the FDA will permit an Abbreviated New Drug Application (ANDA) to be submitted. These submissions require less data, but do require proof that the new drug product's pharmacokinetic properties, its bioavailability, and clinical activity is similar to that of the innovator's drug product.

Supplemental New Drug Application (SNDA)

After marketing a drug product, the manufacturer may desire to make some changes in the drug's synthesis, production procedures or manufacturing locations, packaging, labeling, etc. Rather than submit an NDA, the company may submit a Supplemental New Drug Application (SNDA). This abbreviated application permits desired changes to be implemented.

FDA Classification System for New Drugs

During the drug approval process, the FDA classifies new drugs based on their chemical and therapeutic characteristics. Health professionals employ these ratings to assess the potential value of a new drug.

Therapeutic classification

- Type P — Indicates that the drug represents a major therapeutic gain because there are no other effective drugs available for treating a particular illness or because it has significant advantages compared to currently marketed drugs. Drugs classified as Type P are often given a priority review.

- Type S — Indicates that the drug is similar to other drugs on the market. Such drugs will generally undergo a standard review.

> ## Note
> A Type P drug will be reviewed faster than a Type S drug and will, therefore, generally be marketed sooner if approved by the FDA.

Chemical classification

Type 1 — Indicates a new molecular structure, different from existing drugs, that may be used for the same therapeutic purpose. The drug must not be presently marketed in the United States.

Type 2 — Indicates that the drug is a new derivative of a molecular structure already approved in the United States; for example a new salt or ester of an existing drug.

Type 3 — Indicates that the drug is a new formulation of a drug already marketed in the US.

Type 4 — Indicates that the product is a new combination of two or more drugs.

Type 5 — Indicates that a drug is being manufactured by a new company.

Type 6 — Indicates a new therapeutic indication for a drug already approved.

Note

It is probably NOT necessary to memorize the 6 types. Instead, just remember that Type 1 is the best type since you are placing a new, unique drug on the market. Also remember that Type 6 is important since it will increase the sales and use of a drug product already on the market.

To further complicate matters, some drugs are also classified as:

- Type AA — Indicates a drug with potential use for AIDS or HIV- related disease; such drugs are given a fast-track for potential approval.
- Type E — Indicates a drug for a life-threatening or severely debilitating disease; these drugs are also given a priority review and may be used in patients in imminent danger of death.
- Type F — Indicates a drug that has been placed on hold until submitted data has been further validated.
- Type N — Indicates a drug that is being considered for nonprescription status.
- Type V — Indicates a drug being considered for "orphan drug" status.

Orphan Drugs

An orphan drug is one that would be difficult for a company to develop into a product because the cost of the NDA process would exceed the anticipated market sales. Usually these drugs are useful in treating diseases that affect a relatively small patient population.

The Orphan Drug Act of 1983 encourages companies to develop orphan drugs by giving them incentives such as tax relief, exclusive marketing rights, and faster NDA approval.

Sample Questions

1. How many phases of clinical testing must be conducted before a new drug application may be submitted to the FDA?
   (A) 2 (B) 3 (C) 4 (D) 5 (E) 8

2. Phase 1 clinical trials involve subjects that
   (A) are healthy humans without the disease
   (B) lower species of animals
   (C) are primates
   (D) are in a state of disease remission
   (E) have active cases of a disease

3. The prime purpose of phase 1 clinical trials is to evaluate the drug's
   (A) therapeutic index
   (B) safety
   (C) adverse effects in diseased patients
   (D) efficacy in diseased patients
   (E) marketability

4. In which phase of pre-marketing clinical testing is the institutional pharmacist most likely to be involved?
   (A) 1 (B) 3 (C) 5 (D) 6 (E) 8

5. A pharmaceutical company that is attempting to market a generic version of a drug product whose patent has expired will submit to the FDA a(n):
   (A) IND (B) NDA (C) ANDA
   (D) SNDA (E) letter of intent

6. A pharmaceutical company that wishes to lengthen the expiration date of a drug product based upon additional stability data should submit to the FDA a(n):
   (A) IND (B) NDA (C) ANDA
   (D) SNDA (E) letter of intent

7. Post-marketing surveillance of a new drug product is sometimes referred to as the Phase _____ clinical trial.
   (A) 1 (B) 2 (C) 3 (D) 4 (E) 5

8. Which one of the following grades indicates the most significant advancement when new drugs are evaluated for their relative importance?
   (A) Type 1 (B) Type 2 (C) Type 4
   (D) Type 6 (E) type 10

9. An orphan drug is one that has:
   (A) been removed from the market because of toxicity
   (B) has been discontinued because of poor sales
   (C) has special economical incentives for the manufacturer
   (D) has a low therapeutic index
   (E) has been developed and imported from a foreign country

Answers: (1) B (2) A (3) B (4) B (5) C (6) D (7) D (8) A (9) C

Section E

Requirements for Marketed Drug Products

Naming New Drugs

During the research phases of drug development, the pharmaceutical manufacturer probably identified an investigational drug by a code name, such as WIN 2306. This avoids the use of the burdensome, long chemical name. Once the drug nears its final approval, a specific name known as the nonproprietary or generic name must be established. The company may also select a trade name or brand name for the drug to encourage prescriber recognition of that company's specific product.

The responsibility for designating a nonproprietary or generic name for a new drug belongs to the United States Adopted Names Council (USAN). This group is sponsored by the American Medical Association (AMA), American Pharmaceutical Association (APhA), and the United States Pharmacopeial Convention (USPC). A distinctive generic name, proprietary name or USAN is assigned to each new drug based on the following criteria:

- The name should be short, distinctive, and not likely to be confused with other existing names.

- The name should provide some indication of the therapeutic or chemical class to which the drug belongs.

Patent Protection

There are considerable costs and time delays when a company develops a new drug by the submission of an NDA (New Drug Application). In order to allow the company to recover these costs Congress passed an act to guarantee the innovator company a minimum time period for patent protection before generic versions of the drug product could be marketed.

Up to 1984, innovator companies had a 17-year period of exclusive patient rights, including the development period and the FDA review process. The Drug Price Competition and Patent-Term Restoration Act of 1984, also known as the Waxman-Hatch Amendment, represents a compromise affecting major drug manufacturers and generic companies. The major drug manufacturers were granted longer patent protection (up to an extra five years) while the manufacturers of generic drugs were provided with easier access to approval of their drug applications.

National Drug Code (NDC)

The NDC is a numbering system that aids in identifying a drug product. Third party payers also employ NDC numbers to identify products for reimbursement.

The NDC of a specific drug product contains ten digits. For example, a number may be:

1 0 7 4	0 1 2 8	0 4
(manufacturer)	(ID of specific drug)	(ID of package)

Each manufacturer has its own number. Also, each company can establish its own identification number for a specific drug, its strength, and dosage form. That is, one company might designate warfarin 10mg tablets as 0128 and another company's warfarin 10 mg tablets may be assigned the number 0045. The last two digits indicate the package characteristic such as 04 for blister packs or 02 for bottles of 100 tablets.

Newer drug products have either 10 or 11 digit NDC numbers, of which the first five represent the manufacturer and the remaining digits represent the drug and package.

The NDC Directory is a publication that contains listings of NDC numbers and their identity. Other books, such as the Red Book and the Blue Book, as well as many computer programs have NDC numbers and their equivalents listed.

All prescription drugs marketed in the United States must have NDC numbers. While placing the NDC number on the package labeling is not mandatory, most companies do so. The NDC number also does not have to appear on individual dosage units and there is no federal law requiring that NDC numbers appear on prescription labels.

Good Manufacturing Practices (GMP)

Current Good Manufacturing Practices (GMP) is a set of regulations that specify the minimum requirements required to manufacture pharmaceutical products in the US. They are designed to assure safety and quality of pharmaceuticals and compliance with these regulations is a responsibility of pharmaceutical manufacturers.

While there are many requirements under GMP regulations, this material is unlikely to be tested on the MPJE®. Candidates should, however, be aware that manufacturers must be registered with the FDA and they must describe their manufacturing and production processes as part of the NDA process. The FDA inspects drug manufacturer's facilities approximately once every two years to determine compliance with GMPs, unless a prior history of deficiencies requires more frequent visits.

Adulterated Versus Misbranded Drug Products

A drug is considered to be adulterated if it:

- contains in whole or in part any filthy, putrid, or decomposed substance.
- has been prepared, packaged, or held under unsanitary conditions where it may have been contaminated.
- has been manufactured under conditions that do not meet the standards of good manufacturing practices (GMPs).
- contains an unapproved color additive

Prescription Drug Marketing Act 1987 (Dingle Bill)

The Prescription Drug Marketing Act of 1987 was enacted to correct the problem of drug diversion from normal distribution channels. It includes provisions that:

- require proper storage of drugs and the maintenance of appropriate distribution records.

- prohibit companies from shipping drugs between states without being registered in the state from which they are being shipped.

- prohibit drugs from being re-imported into the United States except by the manufacturer of said drugs.

- require state licensing of drug wholesalers.

- restrict the sale, purchase or trade of prescription drug samples and bars retail pharmacies from receiving any prescription drug samples. Drug samples obtained by a practitioner may not be delivered to a retail pharmacy, even if they are to be dispensed to that practitioner's patients. In other words, a retail pharmacy may NOT possess any prescription drug samples obtained from ANY source. Possession of such samples would be considered to be drug diversion by the FDA.

- Indicate that hospital or health care pharmacies may receive prescription drug samples only if a licensed prescriber has requested them and if precise records are maintained of their disposition. If such samples are received by the pharmacy, they must be stored separately from the normal drug stock.

- prohibit drugs from being resold by hospitals or other health care facilities if they were purchased at special prices. This prevents a hospital from purchasing 1000 packages of an antibiotic at a low price then selling a number of them to a community or chain pharmacy in order to make a profit.

- restrict resale of drug products by hospitals or health care facilities.

- permit practitioners licensed to prescribe to receive drug samples provided that a written request is made with their name, address, medical specialty, signature, name of drug, quantity, manufacturer, and date of request. Drug manufacturers and distributors must keep copies of all requests and keep receipts for three years.

- require sales representatives to be responsible for all samples and take an annual inventory.

- establish stiff penalties for violation of this law.

Product Labeling

The term "label" refers to written, printed, or graphic matter appearing on the immediate container of a drug product. If there is an outside package, any word, statement, or other information present on the immediate container must also appear on the outside package.

The term "labeling" refers to either:

- The information printed on the label and outside package of a drug product. It refers to all labels and other written, printed, or graphic matter either on the product, its container, its wrapper, or accompanying the product. Thus the prescription drug product insert is considered part of the labeling.

- The information printed by the pharmacist on the prescription label for a drug product being dispensed. (NOTE: The prescription label will be discussed later)

While the original Food, Drug, and Cosmetic Act of 1938 specified that all drug products had to be labeled with "adequate directions for use", the Durham-Humphrey Amendment of 1951 clarified these requirements. It states that drugs do NOT have to have adequate directions for use IF they are intended for dispensing by pharmacists, provided that they contain the legend "Caution: Federal law prohibits dispensing without a prescription". In 1997 this required statement was simplified to read "Rx Only".

Labeling Requirements for Manufacturer's Containers of Prescription Drugs

Federal law requires that the following information appear on manufacturer's containers of drug products:

- Name and address of the manufacturer, packer, or distributor.

- Established name of the drug or drug product.

- The net quantity (weight, quantity, or dosage units) in the package.

- The weight of active ingredient contained in each dosage unit (e.g. 10mg or 2mg/5mL).

- The federal legend "Caution: Federal law prohibits dispensing without a prescription" or the more recent version, "Rx only"

- If dosage units are not taken orally, the specific route or routes of administration must be stated (e.g. for IM or subcutaneous injection).

- Special storage directions, if appropriate.

- Manufacturer's control number.

- The expiration date established by the manufacturer.

If these labeling guidelines are not meticulously adhered to, the product may be considered misbranded. Label errors or omissions that would be considered to be misbranding include:

- A false or misleading label.

- A missing name and location of the manufacturer, packer, or distributor.

- The quantity of the container contents is not present. This could be a numerical count (e.g. 100 tablets), net weight (e.g. 50 g) or net volume (e.g. 4 fl. oz).

- All required information is not prominently displayed so that it can easily be read. This includes the listing of officially designated names of all ingredients.

- Adequate directions for use and appropriate warnings to protect those who use the medication (this applies to nonprescription drugs).

Note

The term "adequate directions for use" in federal laws dealing with OTC labeling means that sufficient information is provided on the labeling so that a layperson could use the product safely.

Package Inserts

Besides the above information, the manufacturer is also required to provide a package insert in prescription drug packages. The information in the package insert must be approved by the FDA and is for informational use only, not for promotional use. The following is required to be included in the package insert:

- Description of the drug (including its solubility, chemical characteristics, etc.)
- Clinical pharmacology
- Indications and usage
- Contraindications
- Warnings
- Precautions
- Adverse reactions
- Potential for abuse or patient dependency
- Symptoms and treatment of overdose
- Dosage and administration

- Available dosage forms of the product
- Date of the most recent revision of the labeling
- Recommended or usual dosage

Identification of Commercial Solid Dosage Forms

The Code of Federal Regulations (CFR) requires manufacturers to imprint solid oral dosage forms, whether they are prescription or nonprescription products. The imprint code must permit the identification of both the manufacturer and the specific drug product. There are some exemptions to this requirement. For example, it is impractical to imprint nitroglycerin sublingual tablets.

Sample Questions

1. Which of the following commercial products intended for oral intake must have identification codes on individual dosage units?
   I. Nonprescription tablet products
   II. Prescription tablet products
   III. Prescription capsule dosage forms
   (A) I only (B) III only (C) I & II only
   (D) II & III only (E) I, II, & III

2. Which of the following must be imprinted on each commercial oral tablet?
   (A) Name of the manufacturer
   (B) Name and strength of the drug
   (C) A code identifying each of the above
   (D) The expiration date
   (E) Date of manufacturing

3. Which of the following statements concerning the National Drug Codes is(are) true?
   I. The NDC number must be imprinted on all commercial tablets.
   II. The NDC number on a drug package indicates that the drug has an approved new drug application on file.
   III. The NDC number is used for reimbursement purposes.

   (A) I only (B) III only (C) I & II only
   (D) II & III only (E) I, II, & III

4. A specific drug product has a NDC of 0137-0145-10. The 10 in this designation may represent:
   (A) the generic name of the drug
   (B) the location of the company
   (C) the name of the company
   (D) the trade name of the drug
   (E) a unit dose package

5. Manufacturers will place NDC's on the package labels for:
   I. capsules
   II. oral suspensions
   III. vials of a parenteral solution

   (A) I only (B) III only (C) I & II only
   (D) II & III only (E) I, II, & III

Answers: (1) E (2) C (3) B (4) E (5) E

Pregnancy Warnings

Package inserts generally include pregnancy warnings as part of the "Warnings" section of the insert. Pregnancy warnings are based on five FDA pregnancy categories. These include

- **Category A** - Indicates that there have been adequate, well-controlled studies in pregnant women that demonstrate no risk to the fetus during the first trimester of pregnancy or during the last two trimesters.

- **Category B** - While adequate, well-controlled studies have not been conducted in pregnant women, animal reproduction studies have failed to demonstrate a risk to the fetus.

- **Category C** - The safety of the drug during human pregnancy has not been determined. Animal studies are either positive for fetal risk or have not been conducted. The drug should not be used in human females unless the potential benefit outweighs the potential risk to the fetus.

- **Category D** - There has been positive evidence of risk to the human fetus mainly based upon adverse reaction data from either investigational or marketing experiences. The drug should be administered only if the potential benefits from the use of the drug in pregnant women may be acceptable despite its potential risks.

- **Category X** - Studies in animals, or reports in pregnant women, indicate that the risk of damage caused by the drug clearly outweighs any possible benefit.

Drugs in category X should be considered to be contraindicated in pregnant women or, in most instances, for any woman of childbearing age unless appropriate contraceptive methods are being used. Among the drugs with a Category X rating are Accutane, Cytotec, Thalomid and most "statin" drugs used to reduce serum lipid levels.

The STEPS Program for Thalidomide (Thalomid)

The FDA has established guidelines that a drug company must satisfy in order to distribute a drug that has special safety concerns. Thalidomide is a drug that has historically caused serious teratogenic malformations and was removed from the market in the early 1960's.

Because of new therapeutic indications, Celene has recently re-introduced the drug. This company developed the System for Thalidomide Education and Prescribing Safety (STEPS) to minimize fetal exposure to the drug. Among the elements of this system are:

- Females must undergo pregnancy testing and use effective birth control when being treated with the drug.
- Males must use condoms when having sexual relations.
- All prescribers and pharmacies must be registered in order to prescribe or dispense the drug
- Use of the drug is monitored by mandatory patient surveys that are sent to a quality assurance committee.

Pharmacies dispensing the drug are limited to prescriptions of up to a 28-day supply with no refills. Written prescriptions must be filled within 7 days of being written.

Unapproved Use of Drugs

Can a pharmacist advise a physician regarding the unapproved use or dosage of a drug? Yes! The FDA does not consider prescribing and dispensing drugs for unapproved uses or dosages illegal. Federal law prohibits anyone in the chain of distribution from suggesting to a patient or prescriber that an approved drug may be used for an unapproved purpose. This means that a drug manufacturer cannot promote a drug for a purpose for which it is not indicated. However, the pharmacist may provide drug information upon the request of a physician. If a physician wishes to study the safety and efficacy of a drug for an unapproved indication, he/she should contact the FDA and file a Notice of Claimed Investigational Exemption for a New Drug [IND]. The designation, "off-label use", is sometimes used in place of "unapproved use".

Unit-dose Packaging and Labeling

Many pharmaceutical manufacturers provide their products, especially oral solid dosage forms such as capsules and tablets, in unit-dose packages. These strip packages are convenient for hospital use when daily supplies of the drug for individual patients are sent from the pharmacy to the nursing floors. Because of the small size of these packages, the FDA has issued guidelines as to what information should be on each unit-dose package. This information includes:

- Generic name and trade name, if appropriate

- Amount of active drug or drugs present (and number of dosage units if more than one)
- Name of the manufacturer, packer, or distributor
- The repackager's lot number
- Expiration date
- Any other appropriate information concerning the specific drug (e.g. special storage requirements.)

Many institutions, especially hospitals, repackage drug products into single dose units. A new expiration date must be provided for the repackaged product since the drug product has been transferred from the manufacturer's container, upon which its original expiration date was provided. Calculations for an appropriate expiration date will be considered later.

The return of unused unit-dose packages to the pharmacy for future dispensing is another issue that must be considered. Most states have established their own regulations. Some allow the return of unit dose packages only if originally dispensed to patients within the hospital setting or in some cases by a community pharmacy to a nursing home.

The expiration-dating requirement for a repackaged unit-dose package is fairly strict. While individual state guidelines may vary, the USP/NF states: "in the absence of stability data to the contrary, the expiration date should not exceed 25% of the remaining time between the date of repackaging and the original expiration date OR a six month dating from the date the drug was repackaged, whichever of these two is the LEAST."

Note

The above requirement is stricter than the general requirement in the USP/NF that multiple-unit containers have an expiration date not longer than the expiration date or one year from the date dispensed, whichever is less.

Customized Patient Med Paks

With the consent of the patient, the patient's caregiver, or the prescriber, some pharmacies are providing a customized patient medication package (Med Paks). This package may contain several solid oral dosage forms with directions that specifically indicate the day and time or period of time that the contents of each container are to be taken. The usual information for unit dose packages is needed plus a serial number for the patient Med Pak in addition to the prescription serial numbers for each drug product.

The expiration dating for the Med Pak is based upon the "beyond-use" dating principle but should not be more than 60 days from the date that the Med Pak was prepared.

The MedWatch Program

MedWatch, the FDA Medical Products Reporting Program, is an initiative designed to

- educate all health professionals about the critical importance of being aware of, monitoring for, and reporting adverse events and problems to FDA and/or the manufacturer.

- ensure that new safety information is rapidly communicated to the medical community thereby improving patient care.

The purpose of the MedWatch program is to enhance the effectiveness of post-marketing surveillance of medical products as they are used in clinical practice and to rapidly identify significant health hazards associated with these products.

The MedWatch program has four goals:

- To increase awareness of drug- and device-induced disease

- To clarify what should (and should not) be reported to the agency.

- To make it easier to report problems by operating a single system for health professionals to report adverse events and product problems to the agency.

- To provide regular feedback to the health care community about safety issues involving medical products

Health professionals may report serious adverse events and product problems with all medical products to MedWatch by mail, phone, fax, or over the Internet. A sample of the MedWatch reporting form is depicted on Page 58.

MEDWATCH

THE FDA MEDICAL PRODUCTS REPORTING PROGRAM

For VOLUNTARY reporting by health professionals of adverse events and product problems

Page ___ of ___

Form Approved: OMB No. 0910-0291 Expires: 01-31-01 See OMB statement on reverse

FDA Use Only

Triage unit sequence #

PLEASE TYPE OR USE BLACK INK

A. Patient information

1. Patient identifier — In confidence
2. Age at time of event: or Date of birth:
3. Sex ☐ female ☐ male
4. Weight ___ lbs or ___ kgs

B. Adverse event or product problem

1. ☐ Adverse event and/or ☐ Product problem (e.g., defects/malfunctions)
2. Outcomes attributed to adverse event (check all that apply)
   - ☐ death ______ (mo/day/yr)
   - ☐ life-threatening
   - ☐ hospitalization – initial or prolonged
   - ☐ disability
   - ☐ congenital anomaly
   - ☐ required intervention to prevent permanent impairment/damage
   - ☐ other: ______
3. Date of event (mo/day/yr)
4. Date of this report (mo/day/yr)
5. Describe event or problem
6. Relevant tests/laboratory data, including dates
7. Other relevant history, including preexisting medical conditions (e.g., allergies, race, pregnancy, smoking and alcohol use, hepatic/renal dysfunction, etc.)

C. Suspect medication(s)

1. Name (give labeled strength & mfr/labeler, if known) #1 #2
2. Dose, frequency & route used #1 #2
3. Therapy dates (if unknown, give duration) from/to (or best estimate) #1 #2
4. Diagnosis for use (indication) #1 #2
5. Event abated after use stopped or dose reduced
   - #1 ☐ yes ☐ no ☐ doesn't apply
   - #2 ☐ yes ☐ no ☐ doesn't apply
6. Lot # (if known) #1 #2
7. Exp. date (if known) #1 #2
8. Event reappeared after reintroduction
   - #1 ☐ yes ☐ no ☐ doesn't apply
   - #2 ☐ yes ☐ no ☐ doesn't apply
9. NDC # (for product problems only) - -
10. Concomitant medical products and therapy dates (exclude treatment of event)

D. Suspect medical device

1. Brand name
2. Type of device
3. Manufacturer name & address
4. Operator of device
   - ☐ health professional
   - ☐ lay user/patient
   - ☐ other: ______
5. Expiration date (mo/day/yr)
6. model # ______ catalog # ______ serial # ______ lot # ______ other # ______
7. If implanted, give date (mo/day/yr)
8. If explanted, give date (mo/day/yr)
9. Device available for evaluation? (Do not send to FDA) ☐ yes ☐ no ☐ returned to manufacturer on ______ (mo/day/yr)
10. Concomitant medical products and therapy dates (exclude treatment of event)

E. Reporter (see confidentiality section on back)

1. Name & address — phone #
2. Health professional? ☐ yes ☐ no
3. Occupation
4. Also reported to
   - ☐ manufacturer
   - ☐ user facility
   - ☐ distributor
5. If you do NOT want your identity disclosed to the manufacturer, place an " X " in this box. ☐

FDA

Mail to: MEDWATCH 5600 Fishers Lane Rockville, MD 20852-9787 or FAX to: 1-800-FDA-0178

FDA Form 3500

Submission of a report does not constitute an admission that medical personnel or the product caused or contributed to the event.

Other Product Reporting Initiatives

Other initiatives exist for health professionals and consumers to report problems with drugs and medical devices. These include the following:

MedMARx™

This system was developed by the USP to allow hospitals to anonymously report, track, and benchmark medication error data. It was developed to help reduce medication errors locally and nationally by permitting users to learn from the adverse experiences of others and share the successful solutions and policies that have been instituted.

Medical Device Problems

Health care facilities (e.g., hospitals, nursing homes, etc.), under the Safe Medical Device Act of 1990 (SMDA), are legally required to report suspected medical device related deaths to both FDA and the manufacturer, if known. Serious injuries must be reported to the manufacturer or to FDA, if the manufacturer is unknown. Health professionals within a health care facility should familiarize themselves with their institution's procedures for SMDA reporting.

Vaccine Problems

Adverse events and product problems that occur with vaccines should NOT be reported to the MedWatch program or on the MedWatch form but should be sent to the joint FDA/CDC Vaccine Adverse Event Reporting System (VAERS).

Veterinary Product Problems

Adverse events and product problems that occur with the use of medical products (drugs and devices) in animals should be reported to FDA's Center for Veterinary Medicine at 1-888-FDA-VETS (1-888-332-8387).

Drug Recalls

If a marketed drug product exhibits problems, the manufacturer is encouraged to issue a drug recall notice. Problems may vary from minor problems with a particular manufacturing lot to serious drug-related adverse effects such as a high incidence of hepatotoxicity. Drug recalls are divided into three classes.

- **Class I** The drug product may cause serious, adverse health consequences including death. The recall should include stocks in pharmacies and notification of patients to whom the drug has been dispensed.

- **Class II** The drug product may cause temporary or reversible effects but the probability of serious adverse effects is remote. The recall will usually include stocks in pharmacies.

- **Class III** The drug product unlikely to cause any adverse health consequence.

It is the manufacturer's responsibility to send written recall notices to all wholesalers and pharmacies for recalls in the Class I and II categories. There may be some Class III recalls that are handled with written notices.

It is the pharmacist's responsibility to be aware of all recalls either received in the mail or read in the pharmaceutical literature.

Occasionally, an ingredient present in either a prescription or nonprescription drug product is determined to be potentially dangerous. The FDA may request that a manufacturer of a certain product discontinue sales and/or remove the product from the market. This request for a "voluntary" discontinuation or removal is invariably honored. A recent example of this action was the FDA's request that all companies discontinue marketing products containing PPA (phenylpropranolamine). This was done subsequent to the issuance by the FDA of a public health advisory concerning the risk of hemorrhagic stroke or bleeding into the brain linked to the use of PPA.

Prescription Compounding vs. Manufacturing

With the advent of a multitude of commercial prescription drug products, the pharmaceutical industry has relieved the pharmacist of the need for most prescription compounding. The inherent right of the pharmacist to compound prescriptions has been challenged in recent years mainly due to several unfortunate instances in which pharmacists extended their practice into the area of manufacturing.

The issue is: When does small-scale prescription compounding become manufacturing? The FDA Compliance Policy Guide of 1992 states that pharmacies may compound drugs extemporaneously if:

- the quantity prepared is reasonable for filling either existing prescriptions or those anticipated based upon prescribing habits of prescribers and prescriptions already on file.

- the dosage forms prepared are not being compounded, provided, or sold to other pharmacies or third-parties such as physician's offices.

- the drug products compounded are not ones already available from commercial sources. That is, they are not compounded versions of FDA-approved drug products.

- the ingredients included in a compounded dosage form meet official standards, usually those found in the USP/NF. If a substance does not have an official monograph, it may be used if it is a component or an approved drug product, or it is on a list of approved substances developed by the Secretary of Health and Human Services.

- the pharmacy does not actively solicit business for specific drug products by advertising or by otherwise promoting their compounding capabilities. However, the pharmacy may advertise to both the public and health professionals that it specializes in prescription compounding.

- the pharmacy does not attempt to compound a drug product which is on the list of products that have been withdrawn or removed from the market because they were unsafe or ineffective.

- the pharmacy limits its interstate distribution of compounded products to not more than 5% of the total prescriptions filled by that pharmacy.

May a pharmacist develop a sustained-release drug product similar to a commercial product under his/her prerogative as a compounding pharmacist? The answer is no. This activity is not permissible for several reasons. First, a compounding pharmacist is not allowed to compound drug products that are commercially available. Second, his/her product would be considered a new drug and would require extensive testing including bioavailability testing. Third, preparing a quantity of the product would probably place the operation into the classification of manufacturing, not compounding.

Expiration Dating for Compounded Prescriptions

The pharmacist should base expiration dating or beyond-use date upon the stability information available. In the absence of stability information, the following guidelines are appropriate for beyond-use dating.

- For nonaqueous liquids and solids: not more than 25% of the time remaining on the commercial product or a maximum of 6 months, whichever is less.

- For aqueous solutions made from solids obtained from manufactured drug products: 14 days when stored at a cold temperature.

- For all others: the time duration of therapy but not more than 30 days.

Note

Compounded radiopharmaceuticals and positron emission tomography (P.E.T.) drugs are exempt from the compounding standards.

Sample Questions

1. Which of the following actions is (are) permissible under the FDA rules for prescription compounding by pharmacies?
   I. Advertising to eye doctors that the pharmacy can compound sterile, isotonic ophthalmic solutions.
   II. Sending brochures to nurse practitioners that indicate that the pharmacy compounds topical ointments for the treatment of skin rashes.
   III. Informing an allergy specialist that the pharmacy can compound economical 50 mg diphenhydramine capsules.
   (A) I only (B) III only (C) I & II only
   (D) II & III only (E) I, II, & III

2. A pharmacy begins to receive prescriptions for a capsule mixture that is not available commercially. The usual prescription is for 14 capsules to be taken once a day with two refills. What is the maximum number of capsules the pharmacist may compound under FDA guidelines?
   (A) 14 only (B) 28 only (C) 42 only
   (D) not more than 100
   (E) a sufficient quantity to meet anticipated prescriptions and refills

3. Which of the following may a pharmacy that is specializing in extemporaneous compounding undertake?
   I. advertise and promote with a brochure its compounding services
   II. describe it capabilities to prepare sterile parenteral admixtures
   III. describe dollar savings to customers of a compounded pilocarpine 2% ophthalmic solution

   (A) I only (B) III only (C) I & II only
   (D) II & III only (E) I, II, & III

4. The number of categories of drug recalls is _____ with recall number ____ the most serious.

   (A) 3 and 1 (B) 3 and 3 (C) 4 and 1
   (D) 4 and 4 (E) 5 and 1

Answer: (1) C (2) E (3) C (4) A

Section F

Filling and Dispensing Prescriptions

Whenever the pharmacist encounters a prescription or medication order for a specific drug product, one of his/her first considerations should be whether the drug is classified as a non-controlled prescription drug or as a controlled substance. Most controlled substance regulations are stricter than those for other drug products, particularly with respect to inventory requirements, limits on quantities that may be dispensed and labeling requirements.

Controlled substance regulations will be covered in great detail in Section G of this Guide. In this section the general regulations for the filling and dispensing of prescriptions will be considered, i.e. rules that apply to almost all prescription products.

Federal vs. State regulations

Federal and individual state pharmacy laws sometimes differ. In these instances, the more strict regulation usually predominates and must be followed.

Note

The individuals responsible for the MPJE® are careful to avoid questions that fall into the "gray area". That is, those questions concerning areas of pharmacy practice which either have conflicting regulations between the federal and state governments or involve issues that have not been clearly resolved. For example there may be court cases that have not yet been decided regarding conflicting laws. Before a question is accepted as a test item, its worthiness is evaluated by being tested as a sample question on several examinations. As explained previously, always choose the stricter law or regulation when there is a conflict between federal law and state law. The following guidelines may be helpful when answering MPJE® questions.

Authorization to Prescribe

Each state specifies those types of health professionals who may prescribe and set limits of prescribing on prescribers such as nurse practitioners, physician assistants, etc. Questions in this area are usually based on individual state laws.

Health Professionals That Self-prescribe

Can a legitimate prescriber write prescriptions for their own use? Self-prescribing is acceptable in most states, but some have prohibited the self-prescribing of controlled substances.

Pharmacist's Obligation to Fill a Prescription

A pharmacist may refuse to fill any prescription for any one of several reasons including:

- The prescription is a suspected forgery.

- The pharmacist will be violating the law if he/she fills the prescription.

- The drug or drug product is not in stock.

- The pharmacist believes that the drug product may be harmful to the patient.

Prescription Refills

One issue that faces every prescriber and dispenser is whether a specific prescription may be refilled. Controlled substances have tighter limitations as to whether or how often the prescription may be refilled. To refill prescriptions for other drugs, the prescriber must have indicated how many refills he/she wishes the patient to have and/or a time limitation for refills to be obtained. Many states have established stricter limitations, usually a time span of not more than one year. All refills must be indicated on the back of the original prescription or by using another reliable system (e.g. a computer).

If a pharmacist receives a prescription for a nonprescription drug product with specific refill directions he/she is bound to the refill limits, particularly if the dose prescribed is greater than normal or if the drug is a Schedule V controlled substance.

Prescription File Storage Period

Once a prescription has been dispensed, the federal or state law requires pharmacists to maintain the original prescription on file for at least 3 to 5 years.

Labeling of Prescription Drugs

The nature of information that must be on a prescription label depends upon whether the drug is a controlled substance or non-controlled. It also depends on whether an individual state has requirements more stringent than federal guidelines. The FDCA requires that every prescription must be labeled with:

- Name of the patient
- Prescription (serial) number
- Date when the prescription is either written or dispensed (some states require that the date of a refill be used when a prescription is refilled.)
- Directions for use of the drug product by the patient
- Name of the prescriber
- Name and address of the pharmacy
- Any special cautionary statements that may be appropriate.

Note that the above minimum requirements do not mention expiration dating, lot number of the drug product, name of the drug, manufacturer, or strength. This type of information, although valuable, is not required by federal law and is left to the discretion of the individual states.

Expiration Dating vs. Beyond Use Dating

While the term "expiration date" originated with the dating required on manufacturer's containers, the term "beyond-use date" is now used to describe the dating of drug products that are dispensed by pharmacists. The simplest example would be an antibiotic powder, which is being reconstituted with purified water. The traditional "beyond-use" expiration date for the reconstituted antibiotic solution has been 10 days even though the manufacturer's "expiration date" indicated on the container may have been 2 years for the un-reconstituted powder.

The USP has issued guidelines for dispensing pharmacists with regard to beyond-use dating. For oral solid dosage forms, the beyond-use date is somewhat arbitrary depending upon the pharmacist's professional judgment or specific state regulations. In all cases, the beyond-use date may not be greater than the expiration date on the manufacturer's original package. For other dosage forms in multi-dose containers, the beyond-use date must be the shorter of either the manufacturer's expiration date or not more than one year from the date the drug is dispensed.

While regulations dealing with expiration dates for drug products dispensed by prescription are in the hands of the individual states, the FDA specifies that labels for drug products dispensed to nursing homes, intermediate care, and skilled nursing facilities must have beyond-use dating.

Questions concerning expiration dating must be answered carefully since there are several possible scenarios that involve expiration dating. These include:

- **Expiration dating for a commercial drug product as established by the manufacturer**.
  The manufacturer has established this dating for a specific package and a specific product. Most manufacturers indicate the expiration date on the container in terms of month and year. For example, the designation of July 2003 indicates that the manufacturer has data showing that the drug product will remain within USP/NF specifications at least through July 31, 2003.

- **Expiration dating for a unit dose package that has been prepared from a bulk container of a commercial drug product.**
  The re-packager, usually a pharmacist who is supervising the operation, will determine this dating. The current guideline provided in the USP/NF is for repackaged drug products to have the shorter of two potential dates:

  - 6 months maximum or

  - 25% of the time remaining on the original package of bulk drug product.

Many states, however, have established other guidelines by allowing longer dating - as much as one year maximum or 50% of the time remaining on the manufacturer's expiration date, whichever is less. Since the USP is presently reviewing its guidelines, it is unlikely that the MPJE® will have questions on expiration dating for unit-dose packages.

> **Study Tip**
>
> One possible question that could be asked is how the FDA and other inspection bodies classify a unit dose product that does not have an expiration date? The answer is that the product is assumed to be misbranded".

Sample Calculation

Assume that an original drug product had an expiration date of Sept 2002. A pharmacist repackages the product on January 1, 2002 and is using the FDA guidelines of six months maximum or 25% of the time remaining on the original package of bulk drug product.

A six-month maximum will produce a useful product life of January through June and will result in the expiration date of June 2002. The rule using 25% of time remaining will result in the calculation of 25% of the time from the date of repackaging to the manufacturer's expiration date (a total period of nine months. Twenty-five percent of 9 months is 2.25 months, thereby yielding the expiration date of March 7, 2002.

In the above example the March date is shorter than the June date and must be used. Be careful! An answer of March 2002 would be incorrect since that implies an expiration date of March 31, 2002. If the choices of answers are (A) Jan 2002 (B) Feb 2002 (C) Mar 2002 (D) June 2002 (E) Sept 2002, you would have to select (B) as the correct choice. Hopefully the examiners will not be this tricky!

- **Expiration dating for individual prescriptions being dispensed by a pharmacist.**
  There is no federal law concerning this type of dating. Instead, some states have established their own guidelines, usually a one-year maximum.

- **Manufacturer's expiration dating.**

  All pharmaceuticals must have a clearly legible expiration date on the package. The manufacturer establishes the expiration date for a commercial drug product by conducting extensive stability testing of the drug dosage form in the final package. Data is submitted to the FDA to validate the dating, which is usually a time span of several years.

  Most manufacturers indicate the expiration date on the container labeling in terms of month and year. For example, the designation of July 2004 indicates that the manufacturer has data showing that the drug product will remain within USP/NF specifications at least through July 31, 2004. To be more specific, if the official standards for a 100 mg tablet is "not less than 95% of labeled claim", one would expect that on July 31st, the active amount of drug in the tablet would not be less than 95 mg.

  Pharmacists may not continue to dispense a drug product once its expiration date has passed. Most states require the pharmacist to remove any expired products from the working stock to an isolated area until the product can either be destroyed or returned to the manufacturer.

Poison Prevention Packaging Act (PPPA)

The purpose of the Poison Prevention Packaging Act (PPPA) of 1970 is to provide special packaging to protect children under the age of 5 years of age from accidental poisoning. Almost all prescription drugs, nonprescription drugs, and household products must have safety closures that prevent access to young children.

Included in these provisions are the following:

- If an OTC product is marketed in several sizes, one package size is not required to have a safety closure. Such products must include on their label a statement indicating that the product is for households without children.

- All new and refilled prescriptions must have a child-resistant closure unless:

  - the prescriber specifies that none is to be used. This may only be specified for each individual prescription, i.e. a physician cannot provide a blanket child-resistant waiver directive.

  - the patient indicates that they do not want such a closure. Patients may ask for a non-child-resistant container for a single prescription or they may provide a "blanket waiver" to the pharmacist, directing him/her to never provide a child-resistant container. In either case, it is advisable to have the patient sign a waiver on the back of prescription and to reconfirm the patient's request on a regular basis.

> **Note**
>
> Pharmacists may not use a single patient request for a non- child-resistant container as justification to dispense future prescriptions in such containers.

- When preparing refills for patients, both parts (body and closure) of plastic container units must be replaced. If the container body is constructed of glass, it may be reused but the plastic closure must be replaced. This is a safety precaution since many plastic closures may lose their child-resistant features after repeated use.

Some drug products are exempt from the PPPA by special request of the manufacturer. Examples include:

- Sublingual nitroglycerin tablets.
- Sublingual and chewable isosorbide dinitrate products in doses of 10 mg or less.
- Aspirin and acetaminophen effervescent tablets or granules.
- Oral contraceptives in memory-aid packages (e.g. dial-packs).
- Potassium supplements in unit dose packaging.
- Sodium fluoride products containing not more than 264 mg of sodium fluoride per package.
- Anhydrous cholestyramine and colestipol packets.
- Products in aerosol containers intended for inhalation therapy

Note

Recent additions to the PPPA include regulations about iron-containing products. These include:

- Products containing 30 mg of elemental iron or more must be packaged in unit dose containers.
- Containers that contain more than 250 mg of elemental iron must be child-resistant.

Some drug products are intended by the pharmaceutical manufacturer to be dispensed in their original containers by the pharmacist. Such units must also meet the requirements of the Poison Prevention Packaging Act (PPPA).

The Consumer Product Safety Commission (CPSC) has revised the testing protocol for child-resistant packaging (CRP). Test panels used to assess such packaging will consist of two groups:

- Children under five years of age.
- Adults 50 to 70 years of age.

This replaces the requirement for an adult panel that was comprised of 18 to 45 year old adults. A package will fail the child-resistant test if more than 20% of the children can open the package in a total of 10 minutes. However, to meet adult-friendly requirements, 90% of a one hundred person adult panel must be able to open and close the package in 5 minutes; and then do so a second time within one minute.

Federal Anti-Tampering Act (1982)

Following several incidences of deliberate tampering of OTC products with poisonous substances, Congress enacted the Federal Anti-Tampering Act in 1982. Provisions of this Act require that tamper-resistant packaging be used for certain select OTC's and cosmetics, particularly those taken orally. The package may feature an indicator or barrier to limit access. If disturbed, some visible evidence of entry will be evident. For example, a simple plastic film seal or a tab around the container closure is sufficient. The product label must indicate that it is a tamper resistant package and should indicate how a consumer can tell if the package has been tampered with.

Note

In answering questions, remember that the tamper-resistant and the poison prevention regulations are different.

Sample Questions

1. Enforcement of the PPPA is basically under the jurisdiction of the:
   (A) Consumer Product Safety Commission (CPSC)
   (B) Federal Trade Commission (FTC)
   (C) Food and Drug Administration (FDA)
   (D) Federal Alcohol, Tobacco and Firearms Agency
   (E) Health Care Financing Administration (HCFA)

2. Permission to not use a poison prevention closure on a prescription may be made by the
   I. patient
   II. prescriber
   III. pharmacist
   (A) I only (B) III only (C) I & II only
   (D) II & III only (E) I, II, & III

3. The Poison Prevention Packaging Act (PPPA) was intended to protect
   I. visually impaired patients
   II. geriatric patients
   III. young children
   (A) I only (B) III only (C) I & II only
   (D) II & III only (E) I, II, & III

4. When refilling a prescription that requires a poison prevention container, the pharmacist must always replace
   - I. the glass container
   - II. the plastic container
   - III. the plastic closure

   (A) I only (B) III only (C) I & II only
   (D) II & III only (E) I, II, & III

5. Original packages of nitroglycerin that are exempt from the requirements of the Poison Prevention Packaging Act include:
   - I. sublingual tablets
   - II. ointments
   - III. oral tablets

   (A) I only (B) III only (C) I & II only
   (D) II & III only (E) I, II, & III

6. In which of the following situations are child-resistant closures not required?
   - I. When a prescriber dispenses a prescription drug directly from his office.
   - II. When a hospital pharmacy is filling a prescription for an outpatient
   - III. When a hospital pharmacy fills a prescription for an inpatient

   (A) I only (B) III only (C) I & II only
   (D) II & III only (E) I, II, & III

7. Which of the following types of drugs do not have to be dispensed in a poison prevention package?
   - (A) analgesic for a child over the age of two
   - (B) analgesic for a child over the age of five
   - (C) analgesic for an adult
   - (D) metered aerosol bronchodilator
   - (E) estrogen tablets for a female over the age of 65

8. Which of the following OTC products must be in a tamper-resistant package?
   I. mouthwash
   II. contact lens solution
   III. insulin
   (A) I only (B) III only (C) I & II only
   (D) II & III only (E) I, II, & III

Answers: (1) A (2) C (3) B (4) D (5) C (6) B (7) D (8) C

Patient Package Inserts (PPIs)

Many potentially dangerous drugs must be dispensed with a Patient Package Insert (PPI). This is a document, written in lay language, intended to educate the client about the proper use and potential dangers inherent in the use of the product accompanying the PPI. PPIs must be provided to patients receiving prescriptions for products such as Accutane, HMG-CoA Reductase Inhibitors (i.e. the "statin" drugs), as well as those receiving estrogen or progesterone-containing products. Patients receiving these drugs must receive a PPI prior to administration of the first dose of the medication and every 30 days thereafter as long as the therapy continues.

These rules apply to all physicians, community pharmacists, and hospital pharmacists who dispense the drugs. It also means that hospital pharmacies must provide patient package inserts to hospitalized patients who are receiving estrogen and progestin containing products such as Premarin, oral contraceptive products, and intrauterine contraceptive devices containing these drugs. This may be done by providing patients with the PPI prior to administering the first dose of such drugs and once every thirty days thereafter. This PPI requirement also applies to patients in long term care facilities such as nursing homes.

Prescribers who dispense prescriptions from their offices are NOT exempt from the requirement of dispensing PPIs.

Medication Guides

As part of an initiative to provide patients with comprehensive information about drugs that have been prescribed for them, the FDA, in 1995, announced the Medication Guide program. This program provides standards for the distribution and quality of written prescription information material or Medication Guides to be dispensed to patients. Such guides would be prepared by drug manufacturers on a voluntary basis and in language easily understood by patients. The Guides would be provided to dispensers, who would be required to provide them to patients.

Drug Product Substitution

The regulations that describe the process of substitution of one drug product for another are within the jurisdiction of individual states. Candidates should carefully review the mechanisms and limitations of substitution for pharmacists in the state(s) in which they are attempting to be licensed.

The premise of simple substitution is to provide a lower cost drug product in place of the drug product prescribed. A key factor in substitution has been the necessity that the originally prescribed drug and the substituted drug products had to be PHARMACEUTICALLY equivalent. That is, each drug product must have the same active ingredient, same dosage form, same route of administration, and be identical in strength or concentration. Pharmaceutically equivalent products may, however, contain different excipients.

The term, THERAPEUTIC equivalence is used to denote drug products that are

- pharmaceutical equivalents AND
- bioequivalent.

Drug products that are considered to be bioequivalent have been clinically evaluated and have been shown to have similar pharmacokinetic properties. That is, a similar ADME pathway. ADME is the acronym for

- Absorption
- Distribution
- Metabolism
- Elimination

Data submitted to the FDA by a manufacturer will include graphs that illustrate that two products containing the same drug have similar blood concentration versus time curves. Most critical in claiming bioequivalence is that two products each produce similar

- time to peak
- peak concentrations
- area under the curve (AUC)

The FDA will generally approve the marketing of competing drug products if they are shown not to present bioequivalence problems or, if they do present a potential problem, they are shown to meet appropriate bioequivalence standards.

A third designation, "pharmaceutical alternatives", refers to drug products that contain the same therapeutic moiety BUT may consist of different

- salts
- esters or complexes
- dosage forms
- strengths

Most states do not allow substitution between pharmaceutical alternatives, so they will not be considered in this Guide.

While simple drug substitution is self-explanatory, the term "therapeutic substitution" is more complex. This term is used when a pharmacy has the right to substitute a different drug for the one designated on the prescription or medical order, without contacting the prescriber (e.g. one cephalosporin drug for another). This practice is generally limited to institutions that utilize a drug formulary.

A committee within the institution (usually the Pharmacy and Therapeutics Committee) generally determines which drug products will be included in the formulary. All participating prescribers agree to abide by the approved therapeutic substitution policies. The intent of the drug formulary is to save the institution money by utilizing more economical drug products in a certain therapeutic area and also by reducing the need for the institution to maintain a large drug inventory.

The term "closed formulary" refers to a formulary where only the drug products listed may be used, while the term "open formulary" is used to describe a formulary that permits some unlisted drug products to be dispensed.

When the prescriber writes or the pharmacist selects a drug product for dispensing, one of the following three types of drug names may be used:

- **Generic name** - This is the single specific name given to a drug by the USAN. Each specific drug structure is given only one generic name in this country. For example, ampicillin denotes a chemical that has a specific chemical structure.

- **Trade name or brand name** - This unique name is selected by a pharmaceutical company for its own brand of a generic drug. For example, Apothecon has selected Polycillin as a trade name for their brand of ampicillin while GlaxoSmithKline has registered the trade name of Totacillin. The purpose of a brand name is to encourage prescribers to prescribe a specific company's product exclusively. Remember that every drug product that has been given a trade name or a brand name still has the same, original generic name as every other drug pro-duct containing the same active ingredient.

Some prescribers will write both the generic name and the manufacturer's name on a prescription (e.g. ampicillin -- Premium Labs). When this occurs, the pharmacist must realize that this is equivalent to writing either a trade name or brand name. In this example, the pharmacist is obligated to dispense Premium Lab's ampicillin product.

A new drug product will often have patent protection for a number of years. Its manufacturer has exclusive rights for marketing the drug product and has likely chosen a trade name for the product. The drug product may be referred to as a "Single Source Product" since no other manufacturer markets the same drug. Once the patent has expired, other companies may submit ANDA's to gain approval for their marketing of the same drug. They may choose to use only the generic name or they may select their own exclusive brand name. When more than one manufacturer has a drug product on the market, the term "Multisource Product" is used.

Since pharmacokinetic data for new drug products are sent to the FDA for review, it is logical that the FDA will supply health professionals with bioequivalence information. A publication containing this information is known as *Approved Drug Products with Therapeutic Equivalence Evaluations*, better known as the "*The Orange Book*". Monthly supplements are issued for *The Orange Book*. There are several other reference sources available for determining the status of a specific drug product. These include:

- *United States Pharmacopeia Dispensing Information (USP/DI) Volume III* plus supplements

- *Facts and Comparisons, Inc. Approved Bioequivalence Codes*

- FDA's Internet Web site: http://www.fda.gov/cder/orange/appendix_b.txt

Whenever an innovator's new drug product is developed and submitted with a New Drug Application (NDA), it becomes the reference standard. Manufacturers interested in marketing a product that attempts to duplicate the innovator's drug product must submit to the FDA an abbreviated new drug application (ANDA).

The bioequivalence of the generic versions of an innovator's drug product must be determined. Based on such testing, generic products are classified in one of two categories:

- **"A" rated products** - Such products are determined to be bioequivalent and are thus "therapeutically equivalent" to the brand name or reference product.

- **"B" rated products** - These are products that are found not to be bioequivalent.

Products that are A-rated may be substituted for one another while B-rated products cannot. Most states, however, limit substitution to interchanges between products that are the same dosage form. That is, one cannot substitute a capsule dosage form with a tablet dosage form or an ointment for a cream. Also, most sustained-release or controlled-release dosage forms are not interchangeable.

To further clarify the meaning of these codes, products assigned the "A" code are generally placed into one of several subcategories that generally designate different dosage forms. These subcategories include:

- **AA** Drug products in conventional dosage forms
- **AN** Solutions and powders for aerosolization
- **AO** Injectable products with oil solvents
- **AP** Injectable solutions
- **AT** Topical products (if they are the same dosage form)

Study Tip

It is probably not necessary to learn these subcategories.

Some drug products identified by the FDA as having actual or potential bioequivalence problems, may be acceptable substitutes if the equivalency problem has been resolved by *in vivo* and/or *in vitro* studies. Such drug products are given an "AB" designation, which signifies that the product meets "necessary bioequivalence requirements".

To summarize, products with similar "A" codes and having the same dosage strength may be substituted for each other while products with "B" codes can not.

Recently the FDA further expanded this code system by designating some AB products as AB1, AB2, AB3, etc. These subcategories are intended to categorize drug products, which previously would not be considered bioequivalent into bioequivalent groups. The best examples of the use of these relatively new subcategories are the transdermal nitroglycerin patches. Originally these were classified as "B" since their release mechanisms varied from product to product. However, they are now classified as follows:

Product	Category
NitroDur transdermal (Key) (the reference standard)	AB1
Minitran Transdermal (3M)	AB1

Product	Category
Transderm-Nitro (Summit) (the reference standard)	AB2
NTG transdermal (Mylan)	AB2

Thus NitroDur and Minitran transdermal systems are considered bioequivalent to each other and the Transderm-Nitro and NTG transdermal systems (Mylan) are considered bioequivalent to one another. However, one cannot substitute Transderm-Nitro for NitroDur, or Minitran for Transderm-Nitro.

Another group of drug products with fairly lenient substitution regulations is the amino acid solutions used for preparing TPN's. These are classified as exceptions to the bioequivalence regulations. Such solutions may vary slightly in composition from one another, but it is unlikely that there would be significant differences in therapeutic activity between them as long as the total percentage of amino acids is the same in each. The pharmacist is permitted to substitute such amino acids solutions relatively freely.

As mentioned previously, the "B" codes are assigned to drug products that the FDA does not currently consider to be therapeutically equivalent to other pharmaceutically equivalent products. Since bioequivalence problems often stem from dosage form problems, codes of BC, BD, BE, BP, BR, BS, BT, BX, and B* are sometimes assigned to such products. The meaning of these is listed below:

- **BC** Extended-release dosage forms (capsules, tablets, injectables)
- **BD** Active ingredients and dosage forms with documented bioequivalence problems
- **BE** Delayed-release oral dosage forms (e.g. enteric coated tablets)
- **BN** Aerosol-nebulizer drug delivery systems

Note

Metered aerosol dosage forms are not to be considered bioequivalent unless the drug products meet an appropriate bioequivalence standard.

- **BP** Active ingredients and dosage forms with potential bioequivalence problems. (e.g. injectable suspensions)
- **BR** Suppositories or enemas that are intended for systemic absorption
- **BS** Products that have drug standard deficiencies (e.g. a drug that contains several active components.
- **BT** Topical products with bioequivalence issues
- **BX** Drug products with insufficient data to determine therapeutic equivalence; also used to denote a drug product likely to lose its FDA approval

Study Tip

Good news! It is unlikely that any question will be asked where you must know the difference between any of the above "B" categories.

What is the status of a drug that is manufactured by the New Drug Application holder (i.e. the innovator) but is being repackaged and/or distributed by another company? Since the original company holding the NDA manufactures it, the product meets all bioequivalence requirements and will thus be considered bioequivalent.

Some drugs and their related drug products marketed before 1938 are not required to be listed in the Orange Book because they have a "Grandfather" exemption. Included in this category are drugs such as ASA with codeine, codeine, digoxin, ephedrine, epinephrine, levothyroxine, morphine, nitroglycerin, phenobarbital, oral potassium chloride preparations, pseudoephedrine, thyroid, and quinine.

In addition, some generic forms of nitroglycerin transdermal systems marketed prior to 1962 are exempt as well. While many of these products had bioavailability data, they did not have appropriate bioequivalence data. Over the past few years, however, many of these multisource products have been listed in the Orange Book because their manufacturers recognize the value of providing substitution information.

Narrow Therapeutic Index Drugs (NTI's)

The term, Narrow Therapeutic Index or Narrow Therapeutic Ratio refers to drugs where the multiple between the minimum toxic concentration and the minimum effective concentration is relatively low (i.e. two or less). Examples of such drugs include digoxin, levothyroxine, lithium, phenytoin, theophylline, valproic acid and warfarin. Some states, but not the federal government, have passed their own regulations limiting the free substitution of different manufacturers' products.

Using the Orange Book

The Orange Book is available in two formats, in hard copy or as the Electronic Orange Book at the FDA Internet website (http://www.fda.gov/cder/ob/). Each source provides interested parties with the opportunity to find and compare therapeutic equivalence (TE) codes for multisource products. The bound edition of the Orange Book is published each year and is regularly updated during each year. The Electronic Orange Book is updated continuously.

Tables I and II are sections taken from the 1999 bound edition of The Orange Book. The right hand column for each drug product listed consists of information of minor concern. It contains a number such as N38744 004 with a date such as Nov 11, 1999 immediately below. The number is an application number and product number while the date represents the final approval date. These values are of little importance to the pharmacist. The most important piece of information for the pharmacist is the bioequivalence status of each drug product. That information is provided just before the company names.

Tables I and II depict information about the tablet forms of the drug verapamil HCl (a generic name). Note that various dosage strengths are listed with their corresponding manufacturers. If a specific manufacturer uses a trade name or brand name, the drug product is listed by that name. Otherwise, just the generic name is listed at the top of the column.

Note that the first oral tablet of verapamil HCl listed is Searle's Calan in 40, 80, and 120 mg strengths, all rated AB. The next product is Knoll's Isoptin in 40, 80, and 120 mg strengths also rated AB. Therefore, substitution between these two bioequivalent TABLET products is possible provided the same strength is used.

Note that the 120 mg Isoptin has a "+" symbol just after the AB. This indicates that this specific drug product was the reference standard used by the FDA for bioequivalence study comparisons.

Next, verapamil tablets manufactured by five different companies are listed. All of these have AB ratings and are therefore interchangeable with either Calan or Isoptin.

VERAPAMIL HYDROCHLORIDE

	TABLET; ORAL		
	CALAN		
AB	SEARLE	**40mg**	N18817 003 FEB 23, 1988
AB		**80mg**	N18817 001 SEPT 10, 1984
AB		**120mg**	N18817 002 SEPT 10, 1984
	ISOPTIN		
AB	KNOLL PHARM	**40mg**	N18593 003 NOV 23, 1987
AB		**80mg**	N18593 001 MAR 08, 1982
AB	+	**120mg**	N18593 002 MAR 08, 1982
	VERAPAMIL HCl		
AB	DANBURY PHARM	**80mg**	N70855 001 SEPT 24, 1986
AB		**120mg**	N70856 001 SEPT 24, 1986
AB	GENEVA PHARM	**40mg**	N73168 001 JULY 31, 1992
AB	GENEVA PHARM	**80mg**	N71423 001 MAY 24, 1988
AB		**120mg**	N71424 001 MAY 25, 1988
AB	LEDERLE	**80mg**	N71880 001 APR 05, 1988
AB		**120mg**	N71881 001 APR 05, 1988
AB	MUTUAL PHARM	**80mg**	N71488 001 JAN 13, 1988
AB		**120mg**	N71489 001 JAN 13, 1988
AB	MYLAN	**80mg**	N71482 001 FEB 15, 1989
AB		**120mg**	N71483 001

Table I - Orange Book (Bound Version) Listings for Verapamil HCl Oral Tablets

Table II depicts the Orange Book listing for the extended-release verapamil tablet product, Covera-HS, manufactured by Searle. Note that this product's status is BC, indicting a lack of bioequivalence. In this case, bioequivalence problems are likely due to the special release system for the product.

	VERAPAMIL HYDROCHLORIDE		
	TABLET, EXTENDED RELEASE; ORAL		
	COVERA-HS		
BC	SEARLE	**180mg**	N20552 001 FEB 26, 1966
BC		**240mg**	N20552 002 FEB 26, 1996

Table II - Orange Book Listing for Covera-HS Tablets

Table III depicts Orange Book listings for extended-release oral tablets marketed by several companies including the trade name product Isoptin SR and three generic brands. All of these products have an AB status indicating that they are considered to be bioequivalent. Knoll's brand is again the reference standard.

	VERAPAMIL HYDROCHLORIDE	
	TABLET, EXTENDED RELEASE; ORAL	
	ISOPTIN SR	
AB +	KNOLL PHARM	**120mg**
AB +		**180mg**
AB +		**240mg**
	VERAPAMIL HCl	
AB	MYLAN	**120mg**
AB		**180mg**
AB		**240mg**
AB	SIDMAK LABS NJ	**240mg**
AB	ZENITH GOLDLINE	**120mg**
AB		**180mg**
AB		**240mg**

Table III - Orange Book Listing for verapamil HCl Extended Release Oral Tablets (last column has been removed)

Table IV depicts Orange Book information concerning extended-release oral dosage forms of diltiazem. The first drug product listed is Cardizem CD extended-release capsules. Since there are BC's in front of each Cardizem's strengths, it is not possible to substitute other diltiazem products for these. However, the next group of extended-release oral capsules has AB designations. They are further designated as AB1's or AB2's. This means that an AB1 drug product is considered to be bioequivalent with another AB1 but not with an AB2 drug product.

		DILTIAZEM HYDROCHLORIDE	
		CAPSULE, EXTENDED RELEASE; ORAL	
		CARDIZEM CD	
BC	+	CARDERM	**120mg**
BC	+		**180mg**
BC	+		**240mg**
BC	+		**300mg**
		CAPSULE, EXTENDED RELEASE; ORAL	
		CARDIZEM SR	
AB1	+	HOECHST MARION RSSL	**60mg**
AB1	+		**90mg**
AB1	+		**120mg**
		DILACOR XR	
AB2	+	WATSON LABS	**120mg**
AB2	+		**180mg**
AB2	+		**240mg**
		DILTIAZEM HCl	
AB2		ANDRX	**120mg**
AB2			**180mg**
AB2			**240mg**
AB1		MYLAN	**60mg**
AB1			**90mg**
AB1			**120mg**
AB2			**120mg**
AB2			**180mg**
AB2			**240mg**

Table IV - Orange Book Listing for Diltiazem HCl Extended-release Capsules (last column has been removed)

For example, a prescriber may write for Dilacor XR 180 mg manufactured by Watson Labs, a product that is classified as an AB2. If the pharmacist must substitute for this product, either Andrx or Mylan's 180 mg capsules may be used but not Hoechst's Cardizem SR, which is AB1 rated. In other words, the AB1 products contain the same or a similar release mechanism or may even be manufactured by the same company under contract.

What if a prescriber writes for Mylan's 120 mg extended release capsule? May a pharmacist use Hoechst's Cardizem SR 120 mg capsule? Yes, provided that it is less expensive than Mylan's product. This again relates to the fact that ALL drug products containing the exact same drug and dosage form share the same generic name. Generic substitution means that any drug product, whether it has a generic name only or has been given a trade name or brand name, may be used as a substitute, IF it is less expensive.

The principles explained above apply to other dosage forms as well. For example, Table V depicts Orange Book listings for phenytoin oral suspension, oral chewable tablets, and injectable solution. Note that both the Parke-Davis and Alpharma brands of phenytoin suspension have the same strength and have AB ratings, with Dilantin-125 as the reference standard. There is only one oral chewable tablet listed. Therefore, no equivalent product is available.

The injectable form of phenytoin sodium has three products listed, all with an AP rating. These are considered bioequivalent with one another. As one would expect, there are less bioequivalence problems with solutions than with tablets or capsules.

Most states originally prohibited or discouraged the substitution of sustained-release, delayed-release, and other dosage forms where there may have been bioequivalence problems. However, in some cases, pharmaceutical companies have submitted data showing bioequivalence. The pharmacist must carefully review the data presented in the Orange Book to ascertain the exact status of a drug product.

		PHENYTOIN	
		SUSPENSION; ORAL	
		DILANTIN-125	
AB	+	PARKE-DAVIS	**125mg/5mL**
		PHENYTOIN	
AB		ALPHARMA	**125mg/5mL**
		TABLET, CHEWABLE; ORAL	
		DILANTIN	
	+	PARKE-DAVIS	
		PHENYTOIN SODIUM	
		DILANTIN	
AP	+	PARKE-DAVIS	**50mg/mL**
		PHENYTOIN	
AP		ELKINS SINN	**50mg/mL**
		PHENYTOIN SODIUM	
AP		ABBOTT	**50mg/mL**

Table V - Orange Book Listings for Phenytoin Products (last column has been removed)

Sample Questions

1. Which of the following designations indicate that drug products of the same strength and dosage form may be interchangeable?
   I. A
   II. AB
   III. B
   (A) I only (B) III only (C) I & II only
   (D) II & III only (E) I, II, & III

2. The Orange Book uses the symbol "+" in a series of similar drug products to indicate:
   (A) a bioequivalence problem
   (B) no bioequivalence problem
   (C) the drug product used as the reference standard
   (D) the least expensive drug product
   (E) the drug product that is preferred by most pharmacists for substitution

Answers: (1) C (2) C

Mailing of Prescription Drugs

There are virtually no restrictions on mailing prescriptions via the United States Postal Service (USPS). At one time controlled substances that were narcotics could not be mailed, but that regulation has been eliminated. The USPS still has regulations that prohibit mailing of poisons or alcohol-containing products that could be considered beverages.

USPS regulations do not apply to commercial shippers such as UPS and FedEx. These private companies may establish their own rules for mailing drug products.

Pharmacists who mail prescriptions, especially controlled substances, should package the prescriptions carefully. Any identification on the outside of the package indicating the presence of a prescription drug should be avoided.

Sample Questions

1. The major objective of the Orange Book is to compare drug products that are:
   I. chemically unique
   II. most economical
   III. multi-source
   (A) I only (B) III only (C) I & II only
   (D) II & III only (E) I, II, & III

2. Colonial Labs is the first to place a new drug product on the market. This product would be described in the Orange Book as:
   I. Code A
   II. B rated
   III. A reference drug product
   (A) I only (B) III only (C) I & II only
   (D) II & III only (E) I, II, & III

3. Certain drug products are exempt from the requirements of demonstrating therapeutic equivalence because of:
   I. the grandfather clause
   II. their use in chemotherapy
   III. their high therapeutic index
   (A) I only (B) III only (C) I & II only
   (D) II & III only (E) I, II, & III

4. Major objectives for developing a formulary include to:
   I. reduce drug inventory
   II. allow therapeutic substitution
   III. give prescribers greater latitude for drug selection
   (A) I only (B) III only (C) I & II only
   (D) II & III only (E) I, II, & III

5. Therapeutic substitution is allowed only if an institution is:
   (A) nonprofit
   (B) for profit
   (C) using a formulary system
   (D) under the supervision of a PharmD
   (E) licensed to do so

6. Drug products with which of the following codes may be substituted for one another?
   I. A　　II. AB　　III. B
   (A) I only　　(B) III only　　(C) I & II only
   (D) II & III only　　(E) I, II, & III

7. Which of the following reference sources contain significant information concerning bioequivalence of drug products?
   I. Orange Book　　II. USP DI　　III. USP/NF
   (A) I only　　(B) III only　　(C) I & II only
   (D) II & III only　　(E) I, II, & III

8. Which of the following volumes of the USP DI contains significant information concerning bioequivalence of drug products?
   I. Volume I　　II. Volume II　　III. Volume III
   (A) I only　　(B) III only　　(C) I & II only
   (D) II & III only　　(E) I, II, & III

Answers: (1) B (2) B (3) A (4) C (5) C (6) C (7) C (8) B

OBRA 90 and Patient Counseling

Portions of OBRA 90 directly impact upon pharmaceutical dispensing and care. The Medicaid Prudent Pharmaceutical Purchasing provisions of this Act, establishes conditions for the federal government to reimburse states for outpatient Medicaid services. In order for a state to receive money for its Medicaid program, it must have a drug use or utilization review (DUR) program. The DUR program must include a prospective component (i.e. one that examines future drug use) and a retrospective program (i.e. one that examines past drug use).

> **Note**
>
> Remember that the Federal Health Care Financing Administration (HCFA) controls and administers Medicare while the individual states administer Medicaid programs.

The prospective DUR is a review of a patient's written medical record and/or his medication profile before dispensing a prescription to the patient. The pharmacist must make a reasonable effort to obtain and update a patient medication profile for every person receiving prescriptions. Minimally, the following information is required in the profile:

- Patient's name, address, telephone number
- Age or date of birth
- The sex of the patient
- Disease state(s) information if known or provided by the patient or their physician

- Any known allergies

- A list of medications previously dispensed

- Pharmacist comments concerning the patient's drug therapy, when appropriate

Patients may refuse to divulge any or all of the above information, but the pharmacist should create or refer to the patient's medication profile and indicate the refusal of the patient to provide information.

When a prescription is presented to the pharmacist, he or she must perform a prospective DUR. This consists of:

- A review of the prescription and patient records for over or under utilization of drugs.

- Checking for therapeutic duplication.

- Checking for incorrect doses or dosing regimens.

- Extending a verbal offering to the client or their representative to personally discuss matters that will enhance or optimize their drug therapy.

A critical portion of OBRA 90 that affects dispensing pharmacists is the requirement that an offer to counsel the patient must be provided. The OBRA 90 legislation specifically provides for patient counseling for Medicaid patients. Since Medicaid is under the jurisdiction of the individual states, each state has the right to establish whether patient counseling will be required for all patients. Most states have taken the realistic stand that all patients should be provided with the opportunity to be counseled. Most state boards of pharmacy have or are in the process of establishing standards of care, which require active verbal offers of counseling, not just a check-off system performed by a clerk.

What type of information must the pharmacist provide if counseling is requested? Federal law does not state how much or what specific information is to be provided by the pharmacist. Instead, pharmacists must use their professional judgement to determine the type and extent of information to provide. Appropriate information could include:

- The name and use of the drug
- The route of administration and duration of the drug therapy
- Any special directions or cautions for taking the drug
- Common adverse effects that may be experienced
- How the patient may evaluate the effectiveness of his/her drug therapy
- How the drug should be stored and when it should be discarded
- Whether the prescription may be refilled
- What the patient should do if a dose is missed

Note

Remember. These are only examples of some of the information that the pharmacist may supply. None of these items is absolutely required and the counseling session could include anything the pharmacist considers necessary. Obviously the pharmacist should always inquire if the patient has further questions.

When does the pharmacist NOT have to counsel a patient? Only if the patient refuses to be counseled.

May a pharmacy intern counsel a patient? The utilization of pharmacy interns to counsel patients is a decision made by each state board of pharmacy. Most have included counseling patients as a function of registered pharmacy interns.

The retrospective drug utilization review is a requirement for individual states. It is not for pharmacies. It is expected that each state will establish a committee consisting of physicians, pharmacists, and other health professionals. This board or committee reviews the use of certain drugs over a period of time to ascertain whether appropriate therapy is being utilized. Obviously, the retrospective DUR is performed after prescriptions have been dispensed and information concerning the prescriptions has been sent to a clearinghouse - usually the state's Medicaid center. The DUR board may recommend that some prescribing habits of physicians be changed. The board may also initiate educational programs for both physicians and pharmacists.

OBRA 90 also established and funded demonstration projects with the intent of evaluating outcomes of patient care and the cost efficiency of pharmacist interventions.

Another objective of the OBRA 90 legislation was to reduce the cost of state Medicaid programs. Pharmaceutical manufacturers are required to offer Medicaid programs the lowest price ("best price") for drug products. If the price being charged is higher than the price charged to any other group, the company must offer a rebate of the difference to the state Medicaid program.

Out-of-state and Foreign Prescriptions

Filling of prescriptions written by prescribers in other states or foreign countries is not a clear legal issue. Most individual states have regulations that define which health professionals may diagnose, treat, dispense, and prescribe. Often the regulations specify that only licensed practitioners may write prescriptions with the understanding that pharmacies will fill only those prescriptions written within the state. However, current practice often entails filling out-of-state prescriptions. The prime consideration is for the pharmacist to establish that both the prescriber and the prescription are legitimate. Using his/her professional judgment, the pharmacist should ascertain the legitimacy of each prescription received.

The federal government has not taken a clear stand on prescriptions written in foreign countries by prescribers who are not licensed in the United States. The power to control such prescriptions has been left mainly to the individual states. Some states, especially those bordering foreign countries or with a large number of foreign visitors, allow the filling of foreign prescriptions. As usual, the pharmacist must use his/her professional judgment in deciding which prescriptions to fill.

A side issue relates to whether a pharmacy may fill a foreign prescription and directly export it to a foreign country. This appears to be legitimate if the prescription is for a reasonable quantity of drug. Conversely, a person in this country can import reasonable supplies of a prescription drug. It should be remembered that prescription drugs must be used under the supervision of a prescriber. In filling foreign prescriptions or mailing drug products to other countries it becomes difficult for the pharmacist to determine whether or not a patient is being properly monitored.

Note

NONE of the above rules apply to controlled substances. Federal regulations require that only practitioners licensed to practice in the United States write prescriptions for controlled substances.

Section G

Controlled Substances

Definitions Related to Controlled Substances

The following definitions are listed in the Controlled Substances Act (CSA). While candidates are not required to write out definitions on the MPJE®, they are expected to be able to understand these terms when they are used in questions. Of particular importance are definitions that include lists of drugs. Candidates should review these lists carefully and be able to identify drugs listed in questions. Candidates should not try to memorize any of these definitions, but review them so they are somewhat familiar.

Act - the Controlled Substances Act and/or the Controlled Substances Import and Export Act.

Administration - the Drug Enforcement Administration.

Administrator - the Administrator of the Drug Enforcement Administration (DEA). The Administrator has been delegated authority under the Act by the Attorney General.

Anabolic steroid - any drug or hormonal substance, chemically and pharmacologically related to testosterone (other than estrogens, progestins, and corticosteroids) that promotes muscle growth, and includes:

(i) Boldenone
(ii) Chlorotestosterone (4-chlortestosterone)
(iii) Clostebol
(iv) Dehydrochlormethyltestosterone
(v) Dihydrotestosterone (4-dihydrotestosterone)
(vi) Drostanolone
(vii) Ethylestrenol
(viii) Fluoxymesterone
(ix) Formebulone (formebolone)
(x) Mesterolone
(xi) Methandienone
(xii) Methandranone
(xiii) Methandriol
(xiv) Methandrostenolone
(xv) Methenolone
(xvi) Methyltestosterone
(xvii) Mibolerone
(xviii) Nandrolone
(xix) Norethandrolone
(xx) Oxandrolone
(xxi) Oxymesterone
(xxii) Oxymetholone
(xxiii) Stanolone
(xxiv) Stanozolol
(xxv) Testolactone
(xxvi) Testosterone
(xxvii) Trenbolone and
(xxviii) Any salt, ester, or isomer of a drug or substance described or listed above, if that salt, ester, or isomer promotes muscle growth. Except such term does not include an anabolic steroid which is expressly intended for administration through implants to cattle or other non-human species and which has been

Steroid CIII Refilled 5X's in 6 mos. Transferred once.

Ø questions about penalties/fines/codes

approved by the Secretary of Health and Human Services for such administration. If any person prescribes, dispenses, or distributes such steroid for human use, such person shall be considered to have prescribed, dispensed, or distributed an anabolic steroid within the meaning of this paragraph.

Study Tip

Most drugs that have anabolic steroid activity have the suffix "androlone" in them. Look for that suffix in questions related to these drugs.

Basic class - as to controlled substances listed in Schedules I and II:

a. Each of the opiates, opium derivatives, hallucinogenic substances, including its isomers, esters, ethers, salts, and salts of isomers, esters, and ethers whenever the existence of such isomers, esters, ethers, and salts is possible within the specific chemical designation, listed in (b), (c), and (d) below.

b. Each of the following substances, whether produced directly or indirectly by extraction from substances of vegetable origin, or independently by means of chemical synthesis, or by a combination of extraction and chemical synthesis:

   1. Opium, including raw opium, opium extracts, opium fluidextracts, powdered opium, granulated opium, deodorized opium and tincture of opium
   2. Apomorphine
   3. Codeine
   4. Etorphine hydrochloride
   5. Ethylmorphine

6. Hydrocodone
7. Hydromorphone
8. Metopon
9. Morphine
10. Oxycodone
11. Oxymorphone
12. Thebaine
13. Mixed alkaloids of opium
14. Cocaine
15. Ecgonine

c. Each of the opiates, including its isomers, esters, ethers, salts, and salts of isomers, esters, and ethers whenever the existence of such isomers, esters, ethers, and salts is possible within the specific chemical designation.

d. Methamphetamine, its salts, isomers, and salts of its isomers.

e. Amphetamine, its salts, optical isomers, and salts of its optical isomers

f. Phenmetrazine and its salts

g. Methylphenidate

h. Each of the substances listed in the CSA having a depressant effect on the central nervous system, including its salts, isomers, and salts of isomers

Note

The term " Basic Class " essentially refers to drugs that are in controlled substance categories I and II.

Chemical mixture - a combination of two or more chemical substances, at least one of which is not a listed chemical. Such term does not include any combination of a listed chemical with another chemical that is present solely as an impurity or which has been created to evade the requirements of the CSA.

Commercial container - any bottle, jar, tube, ampule, or other receptacle in which a substance is held for distribution or dispensing to an ultimate user, or held for distribution or dispensing to an ultimate user. The term commercial container does not include any package liner, package insert or other material kept with or within a commercial container, nor any carton, crate, drum, or other package in which commercial containers are stored or are used for shipment of controlled substances.

Compounder - any person engaging in maintenance or detoxification treatment who also mixes, prepares, packages or changes the dosage form of a narcotic drug listed in Schedules II, III, IV or V for use in maintenance or detoxification treatment by another narcotic treatment program.

Detoxification treatment - the dispensing, for a period of time as specified below, of a narcotic drug or narcotic drugs in decreasing doses to an individual to alleviate adverse physiological or psychological effects as part of their withdrawal from the continuous or sustained use of a narcotic drug. Such programs are intended to bring the individual to a narcotic drug-free state within such period of time. There are two types of detoxification treatment, short-term detoxification treatment and long-term detoxification treatment.

- Short-term detoxification treatment is for a period not in excess of 30 days.

- Long-term detoxification treatment is for a period more than 30 days but not in excess of 180 days.

Dispenser - an individual practitioner, institutional practitioner, pharmacy or pharmacist who dispenses a controlled substance.

Export - taking out or removal of drugs listed in the CSA from the jurisdiction of the United States.

Exporter - includes every person who exports, or who acts as an export broker for exportation of controlled substances listed in any schedule.

Hearing

a. Any hearing held for the granting, denial, revocation, or suspension of a registration.

b. Any hearing held to set quotas for the amount of controlled substance that may be purchased or manufactured

c. Any hearing held for the issuance, amendment, or repeal of any rule issued as part of the Controlled Substances Act.

Import - bringing in or introduction of a controlled substance into either the jurisdiction of the United States or the customs territory of the United States.

Importer - includes every person who imports, or who acts as an import broker for importation of controlled substances listed in any schedule.

Individual practitioner - a physician, dentist, veterinarian, or other individual licensed, registered, or otherwise permitted, by the United States or the jurisdiction in which he/she practices, to dispense a controlled substance in the course of professional practice. This term does not include a pharmacist, a pharmacy, or an institutional practitioner.

Institutional practitioner - a hospital or other entity (other than an individual) licensed, registered, or otherwise permitted, by the United States or the jurisdiction in which it practices, to dispense a controlled substance in the course of professional practice. This term does not include a pharmacy.

Inventory - all stocks of Schedule I or II controlled substances manufactured or otherwise acquired by a registrant, whether in bulk, commercial containers, or contained in pharmaceutical preparations and that are in the possession of the registrant.

Isomer - an optical, positional, or geometric isomer.

Jurisdiction of the United States - the customs territory of the United States, the Virgin Islands, the Canal Zone, Guam, American Samoa, and the Trust Territories of the Pacific Islands.

Label - any display of written, printed, or graphic matter placed upon the commercial container of any controlled substance by its manufacturer.

Labeling - all labels and other written, printed, or graphic matter on any controlled substance or any of its commercial containers or wrappers. This also includes such material that accompanies such a controlled substance.

Listed chemical - any List I chemical or List II chemical. (see below for further clarification)

List I chemical - a chemical that is used in manufacturing a controlled substance both legally and in violation of the CSA.

List II chemical - a chemical, other than a List I chemical that, in addition to legitimate uses, is used in manufacturing a controlled substance in violation of the CSA.

Long Term Care Facility (LTCF) - a nursing home, retirement care, mental care or other facility or institution which provides extended health care to resident patients.

Maintenance treatment - the dispensing, for a period in excess of twenty-one days, of a narcotic drug or narcotic drugs in the treatment of an individual for dependence upon heroin or other morphine-like drug.

Manufacture

- The producing, preparation, propagation, compounding, manufacturing, or processing of a drug or other substance.

- The packaging or repackaging of such substance.

- The labeling or re-labeling of the commercial container of such substance.

This definition does not include the activities of a practitioner who administers, dispenses, prepares, compounds, packages or labels such substance in the course of his/her professional practice.

Mid-level practitioner - an individual practitioner, OTHER than a physician, dentist, veterinarian, or podiatrist, who is licensed, registered, or otherwise permitted by the United States or the jurisdiction in which he/she practices, to dispense a controlled substance in the course of professional practice.

Note

Examples of mid-level practitioners include, but are not limited to, health care providers such as nurse practitioners, nurse midwives, nurse anesthetists, clinical nurse specialists and physician assistants who are authorized to dispense controlled substances by the state in which they practice.

Name - the official, brand, common, chemical or usual name of a substance.

Narcotic drug - any of the following whether produced directly or indirectly by extraction from natural sources, by means of chemical synthesis, or by a combination of the two:

a. Opium, opiates, derivatives of opium and opiates, including their isomers, esters, ethers, salts, and salts of isomers, esters, and ethers. Such term does not include the isoquinoline alkaloids of opium.

b. Poppy straw and concentrate of poppy straw.

c. Coca leaves, ***except*** coca leaves and extracts of coca leaves from which cocaine, ecgonine and derivatives of ecgonine or their salts have been removed.

d. Cocaine, its salts, optical and geometric isomers, and salts of isomers.

e. Ecgonine, its derivatives, their salts, isomers and salts of isomers.

f. Any compound, mixture, or preparation which contains any quantity of any of the substances referred to in this section.

Narcotic treatment program - a program engaged in maintenance and/or detoxification treatment with narcotic drugs.

Net disposal - for a stated period, the quantity of a Schedule I or II controlled substance distributed by the registrant to another person, plus the quantity of that substance used by the registrant in the production of (or converted by the registrant into) another Schedule I or II controlled or noncontrolled substance, plus the quantity of such drugs that are disposed of by the registrant. This quantity is reduced by any Schedule I or II drugs returned to the registrant by any purchaser, and distributed by the registrant to another registered manufacturer.

Pharmacist - any pharmacist licensed by a state to dispense controlled substances, and any other person (e.g., a pharmacy intern) authorized by a state to dispense controlled substances under the supervision of a pharmacist licensed by such state.

Person - any individual, corporation, government or governmental subdivision or agency, business trust, partnership, association, or other legal entity.

Prescription - an order for medication which is dispensed to an ultimate user. This definition does not include an order for medication dispensed for immediate administration to a patient. (e.g., an order to dispense a drug to a bed patient for immediate administration in a hospital is not a prescription.)

Purchaser - any registered person entitled to obtain and execute order forms pursuant to the CSA.

Readily retrievable - records that are kept in such a manner that they can be separated out from all other records in a reasonable time.

Register (registration) - refers only to registration required and permitted by the Controlled Substances Act.

Registrant - any person who is registered under the Controlled Substance Act.

Supplier - any registered person entitled to fill order forms under the Controlled Substances Act.

Registration of Manufacturers, Distributors, and Dispensers of Controlled Substances

Any person required to be registered and who is not registered may apply for registration at any time. No person who must be registered may engage in any activity for which registration is required until the application for registration is granted and the Administrator issues a Certificate of Registration to them.

At the time a retail pharmacy, hospital/clinic, practitioner or teaching institution is first registered, that business activity shall be assigned to a specific month of the year. The expiration date of the registrant will be the last day of the month designated. After the initial registration period, the registration expires 36 months from the initial expiration date.

Applications for Registration

DEA Application Forms 224, 225, and 363, forms used by different registrants to register with DEA, may be obtained in person or by writing to any area office of the DEA. DEA Application Forms 224a, 225a, and 363a (i.e. applications for renewal of a registration) will be mailed to each registered person approximately 60 days before the expiration date of his/her registration.

If a registered person does not receive registration renewal forms within 45 days before the expiration date of his/her registration, he/she must promptly notify DEA and request such forms in writing.

Each application must include all information called for in the form, unless the item is not applicable, in which case this fact shall be indicated.

Each application, attachment, or other document filed as part of an application, must be signed by the

- applicant, if an individual
- by a partner of the applicant, if a partnership

- or by an officer of the applicant, if a corporation, corporate division, association, trust or other entity.

An applicant may authorize one or more individuals, who would not otherwise be authorized to do so, to sign applications for the applicant by filing with the Registration Unit of the DEA a Power of Attorney for each such individual. A person who is authorized to sign registration applications must sign the Power of Attorney. It must also contain the signature of the individual being authorized to sign applications. The power of attorney is valid until revoked by the applicant..

Re-registration

Any person who is registered may apply to be re-registered not more than 60 days before the expiration date of his/her registration. Bulk manufacturers of Schedule I or II controlled substances or importers of Schedule I or II controlled substances may apply to be re-registered not more than 120 days before the expiration date of their registration.

Schedule I Controlled Substances

Drugs classified as Schedule I controlled substances are those that have the following characteristics:

- have a high potential for abuse
- have no currently accepted medical use in treatment in the United States
- lack accepted information on the safety of their use, even under medical supervision

Included in Schedule I are the following drugs or substances:

- Opiates. Unless specifically excepted or unless listed in another schedule, any of the following opiates, including their isomers, esters, ethers, salts, and salts of isomers, esters and ethers:

  (1) Acetyl-alpha-methylfentanyl(N-[1-(1-methyl-2-phenethyl)-4-piperidinyl]-N-phenylacetamide
  (2) Acetylmethadol
  (3) Allylprodine
  (4) Alphacetylmethadol(except levoalphacetylmethadol also known as levo-alpha-acetylmethadol, levomethadyl acetate, or LAAM)
  (5) Alphameprodine
  (6) Alphamethadol
  (7) Alpha-methylfentanyl(N-[1-(alpha-methyl-beta-phenyl)ethyl-4-piperidyl]propionanilide;1-(1-methyl-2-phenyl-ethyl)-4-(N-propanilido) piperidine

  (8) Alpha-methylthiofentanyl(N-[1-methyl-2-(2-thienyl)ethyl-4-piperidinyl]-N-phenyl-propanamide
  (9) Benzethidine
  (10) Betacetylmethadol
  (11) Beta-hydroxyfentanyl(N-[1-(2-hydroxy-2-phenethyl)-4-piperidinyl]-N-phenyl-propanamide
  (12) Beta-hydroxy-3-methylfentanyl(other name: N-[1-(2-hydroxy-2-phenethyl)-3-methyl-4-piperidinyl]-N-phenyl-propanamide
  (13) Betameprodine
  (14) Betamethadol

(15) Betaprodine
(16) Clonitazene
(17) Dextromoramide
(18) Diampromide
(19) Diethylthiambutene
(20) Difenoxin
(21) Dimenoxadol
(22) Dimepheptanol
(23) Dimethylthiambutene
(24) Dioxaphetyl butyrate
(25) Dipipanone
(26) Ethylmethylthiambutene
(27) Etonitazene
(28) Etoxeridine
(29) Furethidine
(30) Hydroxypethidine
(31) Ketobemidone
(32) Levomoramide
(33) Levophenacylmorphan
(34) 3-Methylfentanyl(N-[3-methyl-1-(2-phenylethyl)-4-piperidyl]-N-phenyl-propanamide
(35) 3-methylthiofentanyl(N-[(3-methyl-1-(2-thienyl)ethyl-4-piperidinyl]-N-phenyl-propanamide)
(36) Morpheridine
(37) MPPP(1-methyl-4-phenyl-4-propion-oxy-piperidine
(38) Noracymethadol
(39) Norlevorphanol
(40) Normethadone
(41) Norpipanone
(42) Para-fluorofentanyl(N-(4-fluorophenyl)-N-[1-(2-phenethyl)-4-piperidinyl] propan-amide
(43) PEPAP(1-(-2-phenethyl)-4-phenyl-4-acetoxy-piperidine
(44) Phenadoxone
(45) Phenampromide

(46) Phenomorphan
(47) Phenoperidine
(48) Piritramide
(49) Proheptazine
(50) Properidine
(51) Propiram
(52) Racemoramide
(53) Thiofentanyl(N-phenyl-N-[1-(2-thienyl)ethyl-4-piperidinyl]- propanamide
(54) Tilidine
(55) Trimeperidine

- Opium derivatives. Unless specifically excepted or unless listed in another schedule, any of the following opium derivatives, its salts, isomers, and salts of isomers:

(1) Acetorphine
(2) Acetyldihydrocodeine
(3) Benzylmorphine
(4) Codeine methylbromide
(5) Codeine-N-Oxide
(6) Cyprenorphine
(7) Desomorphine
(8) Dihydromorphine
(9) Drotebanol
(10) Etorphine (except hydrochloride salt)
(11) Heroin
(12) Hydromorphinol
(13) Methyldesorphine
(14) Methyldihydromorphine
(15) Morphine methylbromide
(16) Morphine methylsulfonate
(17) Morphine-N-Oxide
(18) Myrophine
(19) Nicocodeine

(20) Nicomorphine
(21) Normorphine
(22) Pholcodine
(23) Thebacon

- Hallucinogenic substances. Unless specifically excepted or unless listed in another schedule, any material, compound, mixture, or preparation, which contains any quantity of the following hallucinogenic substances, or which contains any of its salts, isomers, and salts of isomers:

(1) alpha-ethyltryptamine(etryptamine; Monase, AET)
(2) 4-bromo-2,5-dimethoxy-amphetamine(4-bromo-2,5-DMA)
(3) 4-bromo-2,5-dimethoxyphenethylamine(2C-B, Nexus)
(4) 2,5-dimethoxyamphetamine (2,5-DMA)
(5) 2,5-dimethoxy-4-ethylamphet-amine (DOET)
(6) 4-methoxyamphetamine paramethoxy-amphetamine, PMA)
(7) 5-methoxy-3,4-mdthylenedioxy-amphetamine
(8) 4-methyl-2,5-dimethoxy-amphetamine("DOM" and "STP")
(9) 3,4-methylenedioxy amphetamine
(10) 3,4-methylenedioxymethamphetamine (MDMA)
(11) 3,4-methylenedioxy-N-ethylamphetamine(N-ethyl MDA, MDE, MDEA)
(12) N-hydroxy-3,4-methylenedioxy-amphetamine (N-hydroxy MDA)
(13) 3,4,5-trimethoxy amphetamine
(14) Bufotenine (mappine)
(15) Diethyltryptamine (DET)
(16) Dimethyltryptamine (DMT)
(17) Ibogaine (Tabernanthe iboga)

(18) Lysergic acid diethylamide (LSD)
(19) Marijuana
(20) Mescaline
(21) Parahexyl (Synhexyl)
(22) Peyote
(23) N-ethyl-3-piperidyl benzilate
(24) N-methyl-3-piperidyl benzilate
(25) Psilocybin
(26) Psilocyn
(27) Tetrahydrocannabinols (THC)
(28) Ethylamine analog of phencyclidine (PCE)
(29) Pyrrolidine analog of phencyclidine (PCPy, PHP)
(30) Thiophene analog of phencyclidine (TPCP, TCP)
(31) 1-[1-(2-thienyl)cyclohexyl]pyrrolidine: (TCPy)

- Depressants. Unless specifically excepted or unless listed in another schedule, any material, compound, mixture, or preparation which contains any quantity of the following substances having a depressant effect on the central nervous system, including its salts, isomers, and salts of isomers.
  (1) gamma-hydroxybutyric acid (GHB, gamma-hydroxybutyrate; 4-hydroxybutyrate; 4-hydroxybutanoic acid)
  (2) Mecloqualone
  (3) Methaqualone

- Stimulants. Unless specifically excepted or unless listed in another schedule, any material, compound, mixture, or preparation which contains any quantity of the following substances having a stimulant effect on the central nervous system, including its salts, isomers, and salts of isomers:
  (1) Aminorex
  (2) Cathinone
  (3) Fenethylline

Quaalude - CI but was Rx.

(4) Methcathinone (AL-464; AL-422; AL-463 and UR1432)
(5) (+/-)cis-4-methylaminorex((+/-)cis-4,5-dihydro-4-methyl-5-phenyl-2-oxazolamine)
(6) N-ethylamphetamine
(7) N,N-dimethylamphetamine

- Temporary listing of substances subject to emergency scheduling. Any material, compound, mixture or preparation which contains any quantity of the following substances:

(1) N-[1-benzyl-4-piperidyl]-N-phenylpropanamide (benzylfentanyl), its optical isomers, salts and salts of isomers
(2) N-[1-(2-thienyl)methyl-4-piperidyl]-N-phenyl-propanamide(thenylfentanyl), its optical isomers, salts and salts of isomers

Study Tip

Do not attempt to memorize this list! Review it a few times and identify drugs that you may be familiar with (e.g. marijuana, LSD, heroin, mescaline). These are the drugs that you will most likely be questioned about.

Schedule II Controlled Substances

Drugs classified as Schedule II controlled substances are those that have the following characteristics:

- have a high potential for abuse
- have currently accepted medical use in treatment in the United States or a currently accepted medical use with severe restrictions

- abuse of the drug or other substance may lead to severe physical or psychological dependence

Included in Schedule II are the following drugs or substances:

- Opium and any salt, compound, derivative, or preparation of opium **excluding** apomorphine, thebaine-derived butorphanol, dextrorphan, nalbuphine, nalme-fene, naloxone, and naltrexone, and their respective salts, **but including** the following:
  (1) Raw opium
  (2) Opium extracts
  (3) Opium fluid
  (4) Powdered opium
  (5) Granulated opium
  (6) Tincture of opium
  (7) Codeine
  (8) Ethylmorphine
  (9) Etorphine hydrochloride
  (11) Hydromorphone
  (10) Hydrocodone
  (12) Metopon
  (13) Morphine
  (14) Oxycodone
  (15) Oxymorphone
  (16) Thebaine

- Any salt, compound, derivative, or preparation thereof, which is chemically equivalent or identical with any of the substances, referred to above, except that these substances shall not include the isoquinoline alkaloids of opium.

- Opium poppy and poppy straw

- Coca leaves and any salt, compound, derivative or preparation of coca leaves (including cocaine and ecgonine and their salts, isomers, derivatives and salts of isomers and derivatives), and any salt, compound, derivative, or preparation thereof which is chemically equivalent or identical with any of these substances, except that the substances do not include de-cocainized coca leaves or extraction of coca leaves that do not contain cocaine or ecgonine.

- Concentrate of poppy straw (the crude extract of poppy straw in either liquid, solid or powder form which contains the phenanthrene alkaloids of the opium poppy

- Opiates. Unless specifically excepted or unless in another schedule any of the following opiates, including its isomers, esters, ethers, salts and salts of isomers, esters and ethers whenever the existence of such isomers, esters, ethers, and salts is possible within the specific chemical designation, dextrorphan and levopropoxyphene excepted:

  (1) Alfentanil
  (2) Alphaprodine
  (3) Anileridine
  (4) Bezitramide
  (5) Bulk dextropropoxyphene (non-dosage forms)
  (6) Carfentanil
  (7) Dihydrocodeine
  (8) Diphenoxylate
  (9) Fentanyl
  (10) Isomethadone
  (11) Levo-alphacetylmethadol(levo-alpha-acetyl-methadol, levomethadyl acetate, LAAM]
  (12) Levomethorphan
  (13) Levorphanol

(14) Metazocine
(15) Methadone
(16) Methadone-Intermediate, 4-cyano-2-dimethyl-amino-4,4-diphenyl butane
(17) Moramide-Intermediate, 2-methyl-3-morpholino-1, 1-diphenylpropane-carboxylic acid
(18) Pethidine (meperidine)
(19) Pethidine-Intermediate-A, 4-cyano-1-methyl-4-phenylpiperidine
(20) Pethidine-Intermediate-B, ethyl-4-phenyl-piperidine-4-carboxylate
(21) Pethidine-Intermediate-C, 1-methyl-4-phenyl-piperidine-4-carboxylic acid
(22) Phenazocine
(23) Piminodine
(24) Racemethorphan
(25) Racemorphan
(26) Remifentanil
(27) Sufentanil

- Stimulants. Unless specifically excepted or unless listed in another schedule, any material, compound, mixture, or preparation which contains any quantity of the following substances having a stimulant effect on the central nervous system:

(1) Amphetamine, its salts, optical isomers, and salts of its optical isomers
(2) Methamphetamine, its salts, isomers, and salts of its isomers
(3) Phenmetrazine and its salts
(4) Methylphenidate

- Depressants. Unless specifically excepted or unless listed in another schedule, any material, compound, mixture, or preparation which contains any quantity of the following substances having a depressant effect on the central nervous system, including its salts, isomers, and salts of isomers.

  (1) Amobarbital
  (2) Glutethimide
  (3) Pentobarbital
  (4) Phencyclidine
  (5) Secobarbital

- Hallucinogenic substances.

  (1) Nabilone

- Immediate precursors. Unless specifically excepted or unless listed in another schedule, any material, compound, mixture, or preparation which contains any quantity of the following substances:

  (1) Immediate precursor to amphetamine and methamphetamine: Phenylacetone

  (2) Immediate precursors to phencyclidine (PCP): 1-phenylcyclohexylamine, 1-piperidinocyclohexanecarbonitrile (PCC)

Study Tip

Carefully review the drugs in Schedule II. While some are quite obscure, many are commonly used and are often a source of questions on licensing exams. Remember that Schedule II includes straight opiates and opioids (e.g. codeine, morphine, meperidine) as well as most amphetamines and many barbiturates.

Schedule III Controlled Substances

Drugs classified as Schedule III controlled substances are those that have the following characteristics:

- Have a potential for abuse less than that of the drugs or other substances in schedules I and II
- Have a currently accepted medical use in treatment in the United States
- Abuse of the drug or other substance may lead to moderate or low physical dependence or high psychological dependence

Included in Schedule III are the following drugs or substances:

- Stimulants. Unless specifically excepted or unless listed in another schedule, any material, compound, mixture, or preparation which contains any quantity of the following substances having a stimulant effect on the central nervous system, including its salts, isomers, and salts of such isomers
  (1) Benzphetamine
  (2) Chlorphentermine
  (3) Clortermine
  (4) Phendimetrazine

- Depressants. Unless specifically excepted or unless listed in another schedule, any material, compound, mixture, or preparation which contains any quantity of the following substances having a depressant effect on the central nervous system:

  (1) Any compound, mixture or preparation containing amobarbital, secobarbital, pentobarbital or any salt

thereof and one or more other active medicinal ingredients that are not listed in any schedule.

(2) Any suppository dosage form containing amobarbital, secobarbital or pentobarbital or any salt of any of these drugs and approved by the Food and Drug Administration for marketing only as a suppository.

> **Note**
>
> Notice that Schedule II barbiturates such as amobarbital, secobarbital, and pentobarbital become Schedule III substances if they are combined with noncontrolled drugs (e.g. aspirin) or if they are in a suppository dosage form.

(3) Any substance which contains any quantity of a derivative of barbituric acid or any salt thereof
(4) Chlorhexadol
(5) Lysergic acid
(6) Lysergic acid amide
(7) Methyprylon
(8) Sulfondiethylmethane
(9) Sulfonethylmethane
(10) Sulfonmethane
(11) Tiletamine and zolazepam (Telazol) or any salt thereof

- Nalorphine

- Narcotic Drugs. Unless specifically excepted or unless listed in another schedule, any material, compound, mixture, or preparation containing any of the following narcotic drugs, or their salts calculated as the free anhydrous base or alkaloid, in limited quantities as set forth below:

(1) Not more than 1.8 grams of codeine per 100 milliliters or not more than 90 milligrams per dosage unit, with an equal or greater quantity of an isoquinoline alkaloid of opium

(2) Not more than 1.8 grams of codeine per 100 milliliters or not more than 90 milligrams per dosage unit, with one or more active, non-narcotic ingredients in recognized therapeutic amounts

(3) Not more than 300 milligrams of dihydrocodeinone (hydrocodone) per 100 milliliters or not more than 15 milligrams per dosage unit, with a fourfold or greater quantity of an isoquinoline alkaloid of opium

(4) Not more than 300 milligrams of dihydrocodeinone (hydrocodone) per 100 milliliters or not more than 15 milligrams per dosage unit, with one or more active non-narcotic ingredients in recognized therapeutic amounts

(5) Not more than 1.8 grams of dihydrocodeine per 100 milliliters or not more than 90 milligrams per dosage unit, with one or more active non-narcotic ingredients in recognized therapeutic amounts

(6) Not more than 300 milligrams of ethylmorphine per 100 milliliters or not more than 15 milligrams per dosage unit, with one or more active, non-narcotic ingredients in recognized therapeutic amounts

(7) Not more than 500 milligrams of opium per 100 milliliters or per 100 grams or not more than 25 milligrams per dosage unit, with one or more ac-

tive, non-narcotic ingredients in recognized therapeutic amounts

(8) Not more than 50 milligrams of morphine per 100 milliliters or per 100 grams, with one or more active, non-narcotic ingredients in recognized therapeutic amounts

> **Study Tip**
>
> Note that with the exception of opium and morphine, quantities of drugs listed in the above section as Schedule III substances are all evenly divisible by 3. This may be helpful if you are asked to determine the Schedule of a compounded product.

- Anabolic steroids. Unless specifically excepted or unless listed in another schedule, any material, compound, mixture, or preparation containing any quantity of anabolic steroids, including their salts, isomers, and salts of isomers

> **Note**
>
> Anabolic steroids are classified in Schedule III by the federal government. Some states may classify them or other Schedule III substances in Schedule II.

Schedule IV Controlled Substances

Drugs classified as schedule IV controlled substances are those that have the following characteristics:

- Have a low potential for abuse relative to the drugs or other substances in schedule III
- Have a currently accepted medical use in treatment in the United States

- Abuse may lead to limited physical or psychological dependence relative to the drugs or other substances in Schedule III

Included in Schedule IV are the following drugs or substances:

- Narcotic drugs. Unless specifically excepted or unless listed in another schedule, any material, compound, mixture, or preparation containing any of the following narcotic drugs, or their salts calculated as the free anhydrous base or alkaloid, in limited quantities as set forth below:

  (1) Not more than 1 milligram of difenoxin and not less than 25 micrograms of atropine sulfate per dosage unit

  (2) Dextropropoxyphene (alpha-(+)-4-dimethylamino-1,2-diphenyl-3-methyl-2-propionoxybutane)

- Depressants. Unless specifically excepted or unless listed in another schedule, any material, compound, mixture, or preparation which contains any quantity of the following substances, including its salts, isomers, and salts of isomers:
  (1) Alprazolam
  (2) Barbital
  (3) Bromazepam
  (4) Camazepam
  (5) Chloral betaine
  (6) Chloral hydrate
  (7) Chlordiazepoxide
  (8) Clobazam
  (9) Clonazepam

(10) Clorazepate
(11) Clotiazepam
(12) Cloxazolam
(13) Delorazepam
(14) Diazepam
(15) Estazolam
(16) Ethchlorvynol
(17) Ethinamate
(18) Ethyl loflazepate
(19) Fludiazepam
(20) Flunitrazepam
(21) Flurazepam
(22) Halazepam
(23) Haloxazolam
(24) Ketazolam
(25) Loprazolam
(26) Lorazepam
(27) Lormetazepam
(28) Mebutamate
(29) Medazepam
(30) Meprobamate
(31) Methohexital
(32) Methylphenobarbital (mephobarbital)
(33) Midazolam
(34) Nimetazepam
(35) Nitrazepam
(36) Nordiazepam
(37) Oxazepam
(38) Oxazolam
(39) Paraldehyde
(40) Petrichloral
(41) Phenobarbital
(42) Pinazepam
(43) Prazepam
(44) Quazepam
(45) Temazepam
(46) Tetrazepam

(47) Triazolam
(48) Zolpidem

Study Tip

Note that most of the drugs in the list above are benzodiazepines and end in the suffixes " azolam" or "azepam". Also, important drugs such as phenobarbital and zolpidem are in this category.

- Fenfluramine. Any material, compound, mixture, or preparation which contains any quantity of fenfluramine including its salts, and salts of such isomers:

- Stimulants. Unless specifically excepted or unless listed in another schedule, any material, compound, mixture, or preparation which contains any quantity of the following substances having a stimulant effect on the central nervous system, including its salts, isomers and salts of isomers:

  (1) Cathine ((+)-norpseudoephedrine)
  (2) Diethylpropion
  (3) Fencamfamin
  (4) Fenproporex
  (5) Mazindol
  (6) Mefenorex
  (7) Modafinil
  (8) Pemoline (including organometallic complexes and chelates thereof)
  (9) Phentermine
  (10) Pipradrol
  (11) Sibutramine
  (12) SPA ((-)-1-dimethylamino- 1,2-diphenylethane)

- Other substances. Unless specifically excepted or unless listed in another schedule, any material, com-

pound, mixture or preparation which contains any quantity of the following substances, including its salts:
(1) Pentazocine
(2) Butorphanol (including its optical isomers)

Schedule V Controlled Substances

Drugs classified as schedule V controlled substances are those that have the following characteristics:

- Have a low potential for abuse relative to the drugs or other substances in schedule IV
- Have a currently accepted medical use in treatment in the United States
- Abuse of the drug or other substance may lead to limited physical or psychological dependence relative to the drugs or other substances in schedule IV

Included in Schedule V are the following drugs or substances:

- Buprenorphine

- Narcotic drugs containing non-narcotic active medicinal ingredients. Any compound, mixture, or preparation containing any of the following narcotic drugs, or their salts calculated as the free anhydrous base or alkaloid, in limited quantities as set forth below, which must include one or more non-narcotic active medicinal ingredients in sufficient proportion to confer upon the compound, mixture, or preparation valuable medicinal qualities other than those possessed by narcotic drugs alone:

(1) Not more than 200 milligrams of codeine per 100 milliliters or per 100 grams.

(2) Not more than 100 milligrams of dihydrocodeine per 100 milliliters or per 100 grams.

200mg/100ml

(3) Not more than 100 milligrams of ethylmorphine per 100 milliliters or per 100 grams.

(4) Not more than 2.5 milligrams of diphenoxylate and not less than 25 micrograms of atropine sulfate per dosage unit.

(5) Not more than 100 milligrams of opium per 100 milliliters or per 100 grams.

(6) Not more than 0.5 milligram of difenoxin and not less than 25 micrograms of atropine sulfate per dosage unit.

Study Tip

Note that all of the quantities listed above are evenly divisible by 5. This is a clue that they are classified in Schedule V.

- Stimulants. Unless specifically exempted or excluded or unless listed in another schedule, any material, compound, mixture, or preparation which contains any quantity of pyrovalerone having a stimulant effect on the central nervous system, including its salts, isomers and salts of isomers.

Excluded (Exempt) Substances

The following non-narcotic substances are excluded from all schedules:

Brand Name	Controlled Substance Ingredient
Theophed	Phenobarbital
Guiaphed Elixir	Phenobarbital
Tedrigen Tablets	Phenobarbital
Choate's Leg Freeze	Chloral hydrate
Tedral Tablets	Phenobarbital
Tedral Elixir	Phenobarbital
Tedral S.A Tablets	Phenobarbital
Tedral Suspension	Phenobarbital
Asma-Ese Tablets	Phenobarbital
Azma-Aids Tablets	Phenobarbital
Benzedrex Inhaler	Propylhexedrine
Bronkolixir Elixir	Phenobarbital
Bronkotabs Tablets	Phenobarbital
Vicks Inhaler	l-Desoxyephedrine
Primatene Tablets	Phenobarbital

Note

Manufacturers may apply to the DEA for exemption of a product from controlled substance status. The exemption may be granted if it appears unlikely that the product can be abused.

Use of DEA Form 222

An order form (DEA Form 222) is required for each sale or transfer) of a schedule I or II controlled substance.

> **Note**
>
> Form 222 is required for purchases, transfer of schedule I and II products from one pharmacy to another, returns to a supplier, etc.

Order forms may be obtained only by persons who are registered to handle controlled substances listed in schedules I and II, and by persons who are registered to export such substances. Persons not registered to handle controlled substances listed in schedule I or II and persons registered only to import controlled substances listed in any schedule are not entitled to obtain order forms.

An order form may be executed only on behalf of the registrant and only if his/her controlled substance registration has not expired or been revoked or suspended.

When an individual applies for a registration, the applicant may indicate on the application form that order forms are needed.

Order Forms (DEA Form 222) are issued in mailing envelopes containing either seven or fourteen forms, each form containing an original, a duplicate, and a triplicate copy (i.e., Copy 1, Copy 2, and Copy 3) (see Figure I).

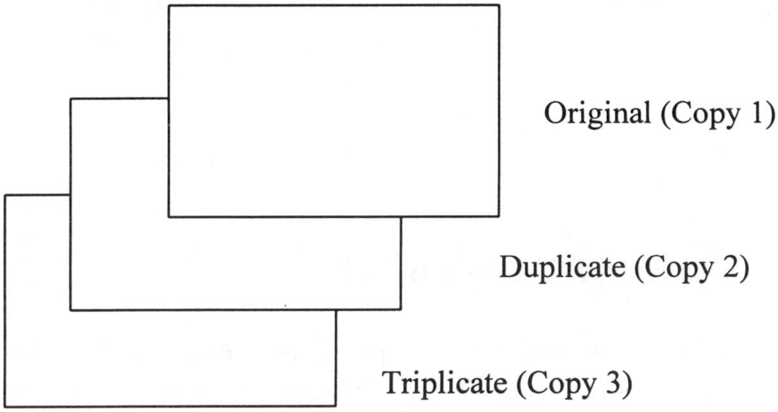

Figure I - Parts of DEA Form 222

A limit, which is based on the business activity of the registrant, is imposed on the number of order forms that are furnished on any requisition unless additional forms are specifically requested and a reasonable need for such additional forms is shown. Additional forms may be requisitioned on DEA Form 222a that is mailed to a registrant approximately 30 days after each shipment of order forms to that registrant. Registrants may also order additional forms by contacting any Division Office or the Registration Unit of the DEA.

All requisition forms (DEA Form 222a) must be submitted to the Registration Unit of the DEA. Each requisition must show the name, address, and registration number of the registrant and the number of books of order forms desired. Each requisition must be signed and dated by the same person who signed the most recent application for registration or for re-registration or by any person authorized to obtain and execute order forms by a Power of Attorney.

Order forms are serially numbered and issued with the name, address and registration number of the registrant, the authorized activity and schedules of the registrant. This information cannot be altered or changed by the registrant; the Registration Unit of the DEA must correct any errors by returning the forms with notification of the error.

Completing DEA Form 222

Order forms must be prepared and executed by the purchaser simultaneously in triplicate by means of interleaved carbon sheets that are part of the DEA Form 222 (see above). Order forms must be prepared by use of a typewriter, pen, or indelible pencil.

Only one item may be entered on each numbered line of the order form. An item consists of one or more commercial or bulk containers of the same finished or bulk form and quantity of the same substance. The number of lines completed must be noted on that form at the bottom of the form, in the space provided. Order forms for carfentanil etorphine hydrochloride, and diprenorphine must contain only these substances.

Note

Remember that when ordering controlled substances on a DEA Form 222, a registrant is not permitted to order different drug products on the SAME LINE. For example, 3 x 100 Percodan tablets may be ordered on one line but not 1 x 100 Percodan and 1 x 100 codeine sulfate 30 mg tablets. Each different product must be ordered on a separate line.

The name and address of the supplier from whom the controlled substances are being ordered must be entered on the form. Only one supplier may be listed on any form.

Each order form must be signed and dated by a person authorized to sign an application for registration. The name of the purchaser, if different from the individual signing the order form, must also be inserted in the signature space.

Unexecuted order forms may be kept and may be executed at a location other than the registered location printed on the form. However, all unused forms must be promptly delivered to the registered site when any federal, state, or local inspector authorized to examine controlled substances, inspects the site.

Any purchaser may authorize one or more individuals to obtain and execute order forms on his/her behalf by creating a Power of Attorney for each such individual. The Power of Attorney must be signed by the same person who signed the most recent application for registration or re-registration and by the individual being given authorization to obtain and execute order forms. The Power of Attorney must be filed with the executed order forms of the purchaser, and must be retained for the same period as any order form bearing the signature of the Attorney. The Power of Attorney must be available for inspection together with other order form records.

Any Power of Attorney may be revoked at any time by executing a Notice of Revocation. This must be signed by the person who signed (or was authorized to sign) the Power of Attorney or by a successor, whoever signed the most recent application for registration or re-registration. It must be filed with the Power of Attorney being revoked. An example of the power of attorney form and notice of revocation is provided on the next page.

Power of Attorney for DEA Order Forms

__________ (Name of registrant) __________ (Address of registrant)
__________ (DEA registration number)

I, ______ (name of person granting power), the undersigned, who is authorized to sign the current application for registration of the above-named registrant under the Controlled Substances Act or Controlled Substances Import and Export Act, have made, constituted, and appointed, and by these presents, do make, constitute, and appoint __________ (name of attorney-in-fact), my true and lawful attorney for me in my name, place, and stead, to execute applications for books of official order forms and to sign such order forms in requisition for Schedule I and II controlled substances, in accordance with section 308 of the Controlled Substances Act (21 U.S.C. 828) and part 1305 of Title 21 of the Code of Federal Regulations. I hereby ratify and confirm all that said attorney shall lawfully do or cause to be done by virtue
hereof.____

(Signature of person granting power)

I, ________ (name of attorney-in-fact), hereby affirm that I am the person named herein as attorney-in-fact and that the signature affixed hereto is my signature.

____

(Signature of attorney-in-fact)

Witnesses:
1. ________________. 2. ________________.

Signed and dated on the ______ day of __________, (year), at ________.

The foregoing power of attorney is hereby revoked by the undersigned, who is authorized to sign the current application for registration of the above-named registrant under the Controlled Substances Act of the Controlled Substances Import and Export Act. Written notice of this revocation has been given to the attorney-in-fact __________ this same day.

____

(Signature of person revoking power)

Witnesses: 1.________________ 2.________________

Signed and dated on the ______ day of __________, (year), at __________.

Filling Orders Written on DEA Form 222

Only a person registered as a manufacturer or distributor of controlled substances listed in Schedule I or II may fill an order form, except for the following:

- A pharmacist who is discontinuing a pharmacy
- If a registrant's registration is expiring without re-registration.
- If a registrant is returning a Schedule I or II substance to the supplier (i.e. wholesaler or manufacturer) from which it was obtained.
- A person registered or authorized to conduct chemical analysis or research with controlled substances may distribute a controlled substance listed in Schedule I or II to another person registered or authorized to do the same.
- A person registered as a compounder of narcotic substances for use at off-site locations in conjunction with a narcotic treatment program at the compounding location may fill orders for narcotic drugs for off-site narcotic treatment programs only.

Note

In summary, any transfer of Schedule I or II drugs from one registrant to another (e.g. pharmacy to pharmacy, pharmacy to wholesaler or manufacturer, etc.) requires the use of a DEA Form 222.

Ordering Controlled Substances Using DEA Form 222

To order a controlled substance in Schedule I or II the purchaser completes DEA Form 222, submits Copy 1 and Copy 2 of the form to the supplier, and retains Copy 3 in his/her own files. The supplier fills the order, and records on Copies 1 and 2 the number of commercial or bulk containers furnished on each item and the date on which such containers are shipped to the purchaser.

If an order cannot be completely filled, it may be partially filled and the balance supplied by additional shipments within 60 days following the date of the order form. The order form is no longer valid after 60 days from the time it was executed by the purchaser.

The controlled substances may only be shipped to the purchaser and to the location printed by the DEA on the order form.

The supplier must retain Copy 1 of the order form for his/her own files and forward Copy 2, at the close of the month during which the order is filled, to the Special Agent in Charge of the DEA office in the area in which the supplier is located.

Study Tip

The person who fills a controlled substance order always keeps the original portion of the order. In this case, the supplier is "filling" the order for the purchaser. When a prescription is filled, the pharmacist is the supplier and therefore keeps the original prescription.

If an order is filled by partial shipments, Copy 2 must be forwarded to the regional DEA office at the close of the month during which the final shipment is made or during which the 60-day validity period expires.

The purchaser (i.e. the pharmacist, physician, etc.) must record on Copy 3 of the order form the number of commercial or bulk containers received on each item and the dates on which such containers are received.

Endorsing an Order Form

An order form made out to any supplier who cannot fill all or a part of the order within the specified time limitation may be endorsed to another supplier for filling.

The endorsement must be made only by the supplier to whom the order form was first made and

- must state (in the spaces provided on the reverse sides of Copies 1 and 2 of the order form) the name and address of the second supplier

- must be signed by a person authorized to obtain and execute order forms on behalf of the first supplier.

The first supplier may not fill any part of an order on an endorsed form.

The second supplier must fill the order, if possible, and ship all substances directly to the purchaser.

Distributions made on endorsed order forms must be reported by the second supplier in the same manner as all other distributions except that where the name of the supplier is requested on the reporting form, the second supplier must record the name, address and registration number of the first supplier.

Unaccepted or Defective Order Forms

An order form must not be filled if it:

- is not complete, legible, or properly prepared, executed, or endorsed; or
- shows any alteration, erasure, or change of any description.

If an order form cannot be filled for any reason, the supplier must return Copies 1 and 2 to the purchaser with a statement as to the reason (e.g., illegible or altered).

A supplier may for any reason refuse to accept any order. If a supplier refuses to accept the order, a statement that the order is not accepted is sufficient. When received by the purchaser, Copies 1 and 2 of the order form and the statement indicating why it was not filled must be attached to Copy 3 and retained in the files of the purchaser.

An order form that is incorrect may not be corrected; in order for the order to be filled, a new order form must replace it.

Lost or Stolen Order Forms

If a purchaser determines that an unfilled order form has been lost, he/she must prepare another form in triplicate. He/she must also prepare a statement containing the serial number and date of the lost form, and stating that the goods covered by the first order form were not received because that order form was lost.

Copy 3 of the second form and a copy of the statement must be retained with Copy 3 of the order form first executed. A copy of the statement must be attached to Copies 1 and 2 of the second order form sent to the supplier. If the supplier to whom it was directed subsequently receives the first order form, the supplier must write "Not accepted" on the face of the form and return Copies 1 and 2 to the purchaser, who must attach it to Copy 3 and the statement.

Whenever any used or unused order forms are stolen or lost (otherwise than in the course of transmission) by any purchaser or supplier, he/she must immediately report the loss to the Special Agent in Charge of the DEA in the Divisional Office responsible for the area in which the registrant is located. The, report must state the serial number of each form stolen or lost. If the theft or loss includes any original order forms received from purchasers and the supplier is unable to state the serial numbers of such order forms, he/she must report the date or approximate date of receipt thereof and the names and addresses of the purchasers.

If an entire book of order forms is lost or stolen, and the purchaser is unable to state the serial numbers of the lost order forms, he/she must report the date or approximate date of issuance of the forms instead. If any unused order form reported stolen or lost is subsequently recovered or found the Special Agent in Charge of the DEA in the Divisional Office responsible for the area in which the registrant is located must immediately be notified.

> **Study Tip**
>
> Carefully review the process of ordering Schedule I and II drugs. An excellent way to review this process is to prepare a simulated, triplicate DEA Form 222 and practice the ordering process, perhaps using a friend as the "supplier".

Storage of Order Forms

The PURCHASER must retain Copy 3 of each order form that has been filled. He/she must also retain in his files all copies of each unaccepted or defective order form and each statement attached thereto. Order forms must be maintained separately from all other records of the registrant.

The SUPPLIER must retain Copy 1 of each order form that he/she has filled.

Order forms and other related documents must be kept available for inspection for a period of 2 years. Illinois Law = 5yrs.

A supplier of carfentanil etorphine hydrochloride and diprenorphine must maintain order forms for these substances separately from all other order forms and records.

On the exam, if not specified, assume Illinois, NOT Federal Law.

Return of Unused Order Forms

If the registration of any purchaser terminates (because the purchaser dies, ceases legal existence, discontinues business or professional practice), or changes the name or address as shown on his registration, or if his/her registration is suspended or revoked, all unused order forms must be returned to the nearest office of the DEA.

Cancellation and Voiding of Order Forms

A purchaser may cancel part or all of an order on an order form by notifying the supplier in writing of such cancellation. The supplier must indicate the cancellation on Copies 1 and 2 of the order form by drawing a line through the canceled items and printing "canceled" in the space provided for number of items shipped.

A supplier may void part or all of an order on an order form by notifying the purchaser in writing of such voiding. The supplier must indicate the voiding in the manner prescribed for cancellation in the previous paragraph.

Persons Entitled To Issue Prescriptions

A prescription for a controlled substance may be issued only by an individual practitioner who is:

- authorized to prescribe controlled substances by the jurisdiction in which he is licensed to practice his profession and
- either registered or exempted from registration pursuant to the CSA.

An employee or agent of the individual practitioner (e.g. a nurse, secretary) may communicate a prescription issued by an individual practitioner to a pharmacist.

Purpose of Issue of Controlled Substances Prescriptions

To be valid, a prescription for a controlled substance must be issued for a legitimate medical purpose by an individual practitioner acting in the usual course of his/her professional practice.

The responsibility for the proper prescribing and dispensing of controlled substances is upon the prescribing practitioner, but a corresponding responsibility rests with the pharmacist who fills the prescription.

An order/prescription that is not issued in the usual course of professional treatment or as part of legitimate and authorized research is not a prescription. A person knowingly filling such an order or prescription, as well as the person issuing it, is in violation of the CSA.

A prescription may not be issued in order for an individual practitioner to obtain controlled substances for the purpose of general dispensing to patients.

Note

If a practitioner wishes to dispense controlled substances to patients, he/she must order them directly from a supplier (i.e. a wholesaler or manufacturer)

A prescription may not be issued for the dispensing of narcotic drugs listed in any schedule for "detoxification treatment" or "maintenance treatment".

Issuing Of Controlled Substance Prescriptions

All prescriptions for controlled substances must be dated and signed on the day when written and must bear:

- the full name and address of the patient
- the drug name, strength, dosage form
- quantity prescribed
- directions for use
- the name, address and registration number (i.e. DEA number) of the practitioner

A practitioner must sign a prescription in the same manner as he/she would sign a check or legal document (e.g., J.H. Smith or John H. Smith).

Each written prescription must be written in ink or indelible (i.e. not erasable) pencil or typewriter and the practitioner must manually sign it.

An agent of the practitioner (e.g. a secretary or nurse) may prepare prescriptions for the practitioner's signature, but the prescribing practitioner is still responsible for assuring that the prescription conforms in all essential respects to the law and regulations. A corresponding liability rests upon the pharmacist who fills a prescription not prepared in proper form.

An individual practitioner exempted from registration under the CSA must instead include on all prescriptions issued by him or her, the registration number of the hospital or other institution and the special internal code number assigned to him or her by the hospital or other institution.

> **Note**
>
> Many states permit institutions such as hospitals to provide prescribers in the institution who do not have their own registration number with the hospital DEA number plus a numerical suffix that specifically identifies the prescriber.

Each written prescription must have the name of the physician stamped, typed, or hand-printed on it, as well as the signature of the physician.

An official exempted from registration under the CSA (e.g. a military or Public Health Service physician) must include his/her branch of service or agency (e.g., "U.S. Army" or ``Public Health Service") and service identification number on all prescriptions issued, instead of the DEA number usually required. The service identification number for a Public Health Service employee is his/her Social Security number. Each prescription must have the name of the officer stamped, typed, or hand-printed on it, as well as the signature of the officer.

Persons Entitled To Fill Controlled Substance Prescriptions

Only a pharmacist, acting in the usual course of his/her professional practice, may fill a prescription for controlled substances. Such a pharmacist must either be registered individually or employed in a registered pharmacy or registered institutional pharmacy.

Detoxification or Maintenance Treatment

In order to administer or dispense (but not prescribe) narcotic drugs listed in any schedule to a narcotic drug-dependent person for "detoxification treatment" or "maintenance treatment" a practitioner must be separately registered with DEA and must comply with the special regulatory standards imposed relative to treatment qualification, security, records and unsupervised use of drugs.

A physician who is not specifically registered to conduct a narcotic treatment program may administer (but not prescribe) narcotic drugs to a person for the purpose of relieving acute withdrawal symptoms, when necessary, while arrangements are being made for referral for treatment. Not more than one day's medication may be administered to the person or for the person's use at one time. Such emergency treatment may be carried out for not more than three days and may not be renewed or extended.

Must be written by an MD.

Schedule II Prescription Requirements

Written Prescriptions and Orders - A pharmacist may normally dispense a Schedule II controlled substance prescription drug only pursuant to a written prescription signed by the practitioner.

An individual practitioner may administer or dispense directly a Schedule II controlled substance in the course of his/her professional practice without a prescription.

An institutional pharmacist or other health care practitioner may administer or dispense directly (but not prescribe):

Valid 7 days.

- a Schedule II controlled substance only pursuant to a written prescription signed by the prescribing practitioner or

- an order for Schedule II medication that is to be dispensed for immediate administration to the ultimate user.

Oral Prescriptions or Orders - In an emergency situation, a pharmacist may dispense a Schedule II controlled substance upon receiving oral authorization of a prescribing practitioner, provided that:

- The quantity prescribed and dispensed is limited to the amount adequate to treat the patient during the emergency period (dispensing beyond the emergency period must be pursuant to a written prescription signed by the prescribing practitioner).

- The prescription must be immediately reduced to writing by the pharmacist and must contain all required information except for the signature of the prescriber.

- If the pharmacist does not know the prescriber, he/she must make a reasonable effort to determine that the oral order is legitimate. Such effort(s) may include a call-back to the prescriber using his/her phone number as listed in the telephone directory and/or other good faith efforts to insure his/her identity

- Within seven (7) days after authorizing an emergency oral prescription, the prescriber must have delivered to the dispensing pharmacist a written prescription for the emergency quantity prescribed. In addition to conforming to the usual requirements for written Schedule II drug prescriptions, this "cover" prescription must have written on its face ``Authorization for Emergency Dispensing," and the date of the oral order. The "cover" prescription may be delivered to the pharmacist in person or by mail. If it is delivered by mail it must be postmarked within the 7-day period. Upon receipt of the "cover" prescription, the dispensing pharmacist is required to attach this prescription to the oral emergency prescription that had earlier been reduced to writing. The pharmacist must notify the nearest DEA office if the prescriber fails to deliver a written prescription to him/her.

What Is An Emergency?

For the purposes of authorizing an oral prescription of a controlled substance listed in Schedule II, the term "emergency situation" means those situations in which the prescriber determines:

- that immediate administration of the controlled substance is necessary, for proper treatment of the intended ultimate user; and

- that no appropriate alternative treatment is available, including administration of a drug which is not a schedule II controlled substance, and

- that it is not reasonably possible for the prescriber to provide a written prescription to be presented to the person dispensing the substance, prior to the dispensing.

Faxing of Schedule II Prescriptions

Faxing of a Schedule II prescription to the dispensing pharmacy by the prescriber or the prescriber's agent is permitted for:

- narcotic substances to be compounded for the direct administration to a patient by parenteral, intravenous, intramuscular, subcutaneous or intraspinal infusion.
- a resident of a Long Term Care Facility (LTCF)
- a patient residing in a hospice certified by or licensed by the state. The practitioner or the practitioner's agent must note on the prescription that the patient is a hospice patient.

In each case, the fax serves as the original written prescription and must be filed accordingly.

The original written, signed prescription must be presented to the pharmacist for review prior to the actual dispensing of the controlled substance. The pharmacist must retain the original fax.

Refilling Schedule II Prescriptions

The refilling of Schedule II prescriptions is prohibited.

Partial Filling Of Schedule II Prescriptions

The partial filling of Schedule II controlled substance prescriptions is permissible. If the pharmacist is unable to supply the full quantity called for in a written or emergency oral prescription, he/she must make a notation of the quantity supplied on the face of the written prescription (or written record of the emergency oral prescription). The remaining portion of the prescription may be filled within 72 hours of the first partial filling. If the remaining portion is not or cannot be filled within the 72-hour period, the pharmacist must notify the prescribing individual practitioner. No further quantity may be supplied beyond 72 hours without a new prescription.

> **Note**
>
> Partial filling of a Schedule II prescription is not permitted if it is being done on the request of the patient (e.g. if a patient only wants half of the medication the prescription calls for). Partial filling is only permitted if the pharmacist is unable to supply the full quantity prescribed (e.g. because he is out of stock).

A prescription for a Schedule II controlled substance written for a patient in a Long Term Care Facility (LTCF) or for a patient with a medical diagnosis documenting a terminal illness may be filled in partial quantities. If there is any question whether a patient may be classified as having a terminal illness, the pharmacist must contact the prescriber prior to partially filling the prescription. Both the pharmacist and the prescriber have a corresponding responsibility to assure that the controlled substance is for a terminally ill patient. The pharmacist must record on the prescription whether the patient is "terminally ill" or an "LTCF patient'.' A prescription that is partially filled and does not contain the notation "terminally ill" or "LTCF patient" is assumed to have been filled in violation of the CSA. For each partial filling, the dispensing pharmacist must record on the BACK of the prescription (or on another appropriate record, uniformly maintained, and readily retrievable) the

- date of the partial filling
- quantity dispensed
- remaining quantity authorized to be dispensed
- identification of the dispensing pharmacist

The total quantity of Schedule II controlled substances dispensed in all partial fillings is not permitted to exceed the total quantity prescribed.

Schedule II prescriptions for patients in a LTCF or patients with a medical diagnosis documenting a terminal illness are valid for a period not to exceed 60 days from the issue date.

Information related to current Schedule II prescriptions for patients in a LTCF or for patients with a medical diagnosis documenting a terminal illness may be maintained in a computerized system if this system has the capability to permit:

- output (display or printout) of the original prescription number, date of issue, identification of prescribing individual practitioner, identification of patient, address of the LTCF or address of the hospital or residence of the patient, identification of medication authorized (to include dosage, form, strength and quantity), listing of the partial fillings that have been dispensed under each prescription and other information required by the CSA.

- Immediate (real-time) updating of the prescription record each time a partial filling of the prescription is conducted.

What can be changed on a CII Rx?

Law → Gray area

DEA - released a statement saying it was ok, but it's not law.

Labeling Schedule II Prescriptions

The pharmacist filling a written or emergency oral prescription for a Schedule II controlled substance must affix to the prescription package a label showing the

- date of filling
- pharmacy name and address
- serial number of the prescription
- name of the patient
- name of the prescribing practitioner
- directions for use
- following warning: "Caution: Federal law prohibits the transfer of this drug to any person other than the patient for whom it was prescribed."

> **Note**
>
> This "Caution" statement is not required to appear on the label of a Schedule II controlled substance dispensed for use in clinical investigations which are" blinded" (e.g. a double-blinded study)

- other cautionary statements, if any, contained in such prescription or required by law

These requirements do not apply when a controlled substance listed in Schedule II is prescribed for administration to a patient in an institution, provided that:

- not more than 7-day supply of the Schedule II controlled substance is dispensed at one time

- the controlled substance listed in Schedule II is not in the possession of the ultimate user prior to the administration

- the institution maintains appropriate safeguards and records regarding the proper administration, control, dispensing, and storage of the controlled substance listed in Schedule II, and

- The system employed by the pharmacist in filling a prescription is adequate to identify the supplier, the product, and the patient, and to set forth the directions for use and cautionary statements, if any, contained in the prescription or required by law.

Schedule III, IV, and V Prescription Requirements

6 mos

A pharmacist may dispense a Schedule III, IV, or V controlled substance prescription drug only pursuant to

- a written prescription signed by a practitioner or

- a fax of a written, signed prescription transmitted by the prescriber or the prescriber's agent to the pharmacy or

- pursuant to an oral prescription made by an individual practitioner and promptly reduced to writing by the pharmacist containing all information required except for the signature of the prescriber.

A prescriber may administer or dispense a Schedule III, IV, or V controlled substance directly to a consumer in the course of his/her professional practice without a prescription.

Illinois: III IV + V's can be faxed.

An institutional practitioner-pharmacist may administer or dispense directly (but not prescribe) a Schedule III, IV, or V controlled substance only pursuant to

- a written prescription signed by a prescriber.

- a fax of a written prescription or order for medication transmitted by the prescriber or the prescriber's agent to the institutional practitioner-pharmacist.

- an oral prescription made by a prescriber and promptly reduced to writing by the pharmacist (containing all required information except for the signature of the prescriber).

- an order for medication made by a prescriber which is dispensed for immediate administration to the ultimate user.

Refilling of Schedule III, IV or V Prescriptions

Prescriptions for Schedule III or IV controlled substances may be refilled not more than five times in a six-month period from the date on which such prescription was issued, if authorized by the prescriber.

A record of each refilling of a prescription must be entered on the back of the prescription or on another appropriate document. If entered on another document, such as a medication record, the document must be uniformly maintained and readily retrievable. The following information must be retrievable by the prescription number:

- name and dosage form of the controlled substance
- date filled or refilled

- quantity dispensed
- initials of the dispensing pharmacist for each refill
- the total number of refills for that prescription

If the pharmacist just initials and dates the back of the prescription it is assumed that the full face amount of the prescription has been dispensed as a refill.

The prescribing practitioner may authorize additional refills of Schedule III or IV controlled substances on the original prescription through an oral refill authorization transmitted to the pharmacist provided the following conditions are met:

- The total quantity authorized, including the amount of the original prescription, does not exceed five refills within a six-month period from the date of issue of the original prescription.

- The pharmacist obtaining the oral authorization must record on the reverse of the original prescription the

    - date of authorization
    - quantity of medication per refill
    - number of additional refills authorized
    - initials of the pharmacist who received the authorization from the prescriber who issued the original prescription.

- The quantity of each additional refill authorized is equal to or less than the quantity authorized for the initial filling of the original prescription.

- The prescriber must issue a new and separate prescription for any additional quantities beyond the five refill, six-month limitation.

As an alternative to the procedures described above, an automated data processing system (i.e. a computer) may be used for the storage and retrieval of refill information for prescription orders for Schedule III and IV controlled substances, subject to the following conditions:

- The computerized system must provide on-line retrieval (via CRT display or hard-copy printout) of original prescription order information for those prescription orders which are currently authorized for refilling. This must include, but is not limited to the:

  - original prescription number
  - date of issuance of the original prescription order by the prescriber
  - full name and address of the patient
  - name, address, and DEA registration number of the prescriber
  - name, strength, dosage form and quantity of the controlled substance prescribed (and quantity dispensed if different from the quantity prescribed)
  - total number of refills authorized by the prescriber

- The computerized system must provide on-line retrieval (via CRT display or hard-copy printout) of the current refill history for Schedule III or IV controlled substance prescription orders (those authorized for refill during the past six months.) This refill history must include, but is not limited to the

  - name of the controlled substance
  - date of refill
  - quantity dispensed
  - identification code, or name or initials of the dispensing pharmacist for each refill

  - total number of refills dispensed to date for that prescription order.

- The individual pharmacist who makes use of such a system must provide documentation of the fact that the refill information entered into the computer each time a pharmacist refills an original prescription order for a Schedule III or IV controlled substance is correct.

- If such a system provides a hard-copy printout of each day's controlled substance prescription order refill data, that printout must be verified, dated, and signed by the individual pharmacist who refilled such a prescription order. The individual pharmacist must verify that the data indicated is correct and then sign this document in the same manner as he would sign a check or legal document (e.g., J. H. Smith, or John H. Smith). This document must be maintained in a separate file at that pharmacy for a period of two years from the dispensing date. This printout of the day's controlled substance prescription order refill data must be provided to each pharmacy using such a computerized system within 72 hours of the date on which the refill was dispensed. It must be verified and signed by each pharmacist who is involved with such dispensing. In lieu of such a printout, the pharmacy must maintain a bound logbook, or separate file, in which each individual pharmacist involved in such dispensing, must sign a statement each day. The statement must attest to the fact that the refill information entered into the computer that day has been reviewed by him/her and is correct as shown. Such a book or file must be maintained at the pharmacy using such a system for a period of two years after the date of dispensing the appropriately authorized refill.

- Any such computerized system must have the capability of producing a printout of any refill data that the user pharmacy is responsible for maintaining under the CSA. For example, this would include a refill-by-refill audit trail for any specified strength and dosage form of any controlled substance (by either brand or generic name or both). Such a printout must include

  - name of the prescriber
  - name and address of the patient
  - quantity dispensed on each refill
  - date of dispensing for each refill
  - name or identification code of the dispensing pharmacist
  - the number of the original prescription order

- In any computerized system employed by a user pharmacy, the central record-keeping location must be capable of sending the printout to the pharmacy within 48 hours.

- In the event that a pharmacy employing such a computerized system experiences system downtime, the pharmacy must have an auxiliary procedure which will be used for documenting refills of Schedule III and IV controlled substance prescription orders. This auxiliary procedure must insure that refills are authorized by the original prescription order, that the maximum number of refills has not been exceeded, and that all of the appropriate data is retained for on-line data entry as soon as the computer system is available for use again.

When filing refill information for original prescription orders for Schedule III or IV controlled substances, a pharmacy may use only one of the two systems described above (i.e. putting it on the back of the original prescription or onto a computerized record-keeping system).

Partial Filling of Schedule III, IV, and V Prescriptions

The partial filling of a prescription for a controlled substance listed in Schedule III, IV, or V is permissible, provided that:

- Each partial filling is recorded in the same manner as a refilling (see above).
- The total quantity dispensed in all partial fillings does not exceed the total quantity prescribed.
- No dispensing occurs beyond 6 months after the date on which the prescription was issued.

Labeling and Filling of Schedule III, IV and V Prescriptions

The pharmacist filling a prescription for a Schedule III, IV, or V controlled substance must affix to the package a label showing the

- pharmacy name and address
- serial number
- date of initial filling
- name of the patient
- name of the practitioner issuing the prescription
- directions for use

- the following warning: "Caution: Federal law prohibits the transfer of this drug to any person other than the patient for whom it was prescribed".

> **Note**
>
> This "Caution" statement is NOT required to appear on the label of a controlled substance in ScheduleV or for any controlled substance dispensed for use in clinical investigations which are "blinded".

- cautionary statements, if any, contained in the prescription, as required by law.

These requirements do not apply when a Schedule III, IV, or V controlled substance is prescribed for administration to an ultimate user who is institutionalized, provided that:

- Not more than a 34-day supply or 100 dosage units, whichever is less, of the controlled substance listed in Schedule III, IV, or V is dispensed at one time

- The controlled substance listed in Schedule III, IV, or V is not in the possession of the ultimate user prior to administration

- The institution maintains appropriate safeguards and records the proper administration, control, dispensing, and storage of the Schedule III, IV, or V controlled substances

- The system employed by the pharmacist in filling a prescription is adequate to identify the supplier, the product and the patient, and to include the directions for use and cautionary statements, if any, contained in the prescription or required by law.

Transfer Between Pharmacies of Prescription Information For Schedules III, IV, and V Controlled Substances For Refill Purposes

Original prescription information for a Schedule III, IV or V controlled substance may be transferred on a one-time basis only for the purpose of refill dispensing.

Must have been dispensed once before transfer.

Pharmacies electronically sharing a real-time, on-line database may transfer up to the maximum refills permitted by law and the prescriber's authorization. Such transfers are subject to the following requirements:

- The transfer is communicated directly between two licensed pharmacists and the transferring pharmacist records the following information:
  - Writes the word ``VOID" on the face of the invalidated prescription.
  - Records on the reverse of the invalidated prescription the name, address and DEA registration number of the pharmacy to which it was transferred and the name of the pharmacist receiving the prescription information.
  - Records the date of the transfer and the name of the pharmacist transferring the information.
- The pharmacist receiving the transferred prescription information must reduce to writing the following:
  - Writes the word “transfer” on the face of the transferred prescription.

Illinois: Retain info for 5 years

Illinois Law: If you have a common electronic database, you can transfer back + fourth. "shared common drive"

- All information required on a prescription by the CSA including the:

    * date of issuance of original prescription

    * original number of refills authorized on the original prescription

    * date of original dispensing

    * number of valid refills remaining

    * date(s) and locations of previous refill(s)

    * pharmacy's name, address, DEA registration number and prescription number from which the prescription information was transferred

    * name of pharmacist who transferred the prescription

    * pharmacy's name, address, DEA registration number and prescription number from which the prescription was originally filled

• The original and transferred prescription(s) must be maintained for a period of two years from the date of last refill.

Pharmacies electronically accessing the same prescription record must satisfy all information requirements as for the transfer of manual prescriptions.

The procedure allowing the transfer of prescription information for refill purposes is permissible only if allowable under existing state or other applicable law.

Dispensing Controlled Substances Without a Prescription

A Schedule II, III, IV, or V controlled substance that is not a prescription drug pursuant to any federal, state or local law may be dispensed by a pharmacist without a prescription to a retail purchaser provided that:

- such dispensing is made only by a pharmacist, and not by a non-pharmacist employee even if under the supervision of a pharmacist (although after the pharmacist has fulfilled his professional and legal responsibilities, the actual cash, credit transaction, or delivery, may be completed by a non-pharmacist)

> **Note**
> Only a pharmacist may dispense an OTC controlled substance, although a non-pharmacist may complete the sale.

- not more than 240 mL (8 ounces) of any such controlled substance containing opium, nor more than 120 mL (4 fluid ounces) of any other such controlled substance nor more than 48 dosage units of any such controlled substance containing opium, nor more than 24 dosage units of any other such controlled substance may be dispensed at retail to the same purchaser in any given 48-hour period

> **Note**
> Therefore, a pharmacist who sells a codeine containing cough preparation over-the-counter may not sell more than 4 fluid ounces to a given purchaser in any 48-hour period.

- the purchaser is at least 18 years of age

- the pharmacist must require every purchaser of a controlled substance not known to him/her to furnish suitable identification (including proof of age where appropriate)

- a bound record book for dispensing of controlled substances without a prescription must be maintained by the pharmacist. The book must contain the

  - name and address of each purchaser

  - name and quantity of controlled substance purchased

  - date of each purchase

  - name or initials of the pharmacist who dispensed the substance to the purchaser

The record book must be maintained as other records described in the CSA

Controlled Substance Records

Prescribers

Prescribers are required to keep records of controlled substances in schedules II, III, IV, and V that are dispensed, other than by prescribing or administering, in their practice. Such practitioners are NOT required to keep records of controlled substances in schedules II, III, IV, and V which are prescribed in the lawful course of their practice, unless such substances are prescribed as part of a maintenance or detoxification treatment of an individual.

Prescribers are not required to keep records of controlled substances listed in Schedules II, III, IV and V that are administered in their practice unless the prescriber regularly engages in the dispensing or administering of controlled substances and charges patients, either separately or together, with charges for other professional services, for substances so dispensed or administered.

Records must be kept for controlled substances administered in the course of maintenance or detoxification treatment of an individual.

Mid-level Practitioners

Each registered mid-level practitioner must maintain, in a readily retrievable manner, those documents required by the state in which he/she practices which describe the conditions and extent of his/her authorization to dispense controlled substances. The practitioner must make such documents available for inspection and copying by authorized employees of the DEA. Examples of such documentation include protocols, practice guidelines or practice agreements.

Pharmacists

Each registered pharmacy must maintain the following inventories and records of controlled substances:

- Inventories and records of all controlled substances listed in Schedules I and II must be maintained separately from all other records of the pharmacy, and prescriptions for such substances must be maintained in a separate prescription file

- Inventories and records of controlled substances listed in Schedules III, IV, and V must be maintained either separately from all other records of the pharmacy or in such form that the information required is readily retrievable from ordinary business records of the pharmacy. Prescriptions for such substances must be maintained either in a separate prescription file for controlled substances listed in Schedules III, IV, and V only or in such form that they are readily retrievable from the other prescription records of the pharmacy.

- Prescriptions will be deemed readily retrievable if, at the time they are initially filed, the face of the prescription is stamped in red ink in the lower right corner with the letter "C" no less than 1 inch high and filed either in the prescription file for controlled substances listed in Schedules I and II or in the usual consecutively numbered prescription file for non-controlled substances.

- If a pharmacy employs an automatic data processing (computer) system or other electronic record-keeping system for prescriptions that permits identification by prescription number and retrieval of original documents by prescriber's name, patient's name, drug dispensed, and date filled, then the requirement to mark the hard copy prescription with a red "C" is waived.

Note

Schedule III, IV, or V prescriptions need NOT be stamped with the red letter "C" if a computer record of these prescriptions is maintained.

Other Entities

Each registered manufacturer, distributor, importer, exporter, narcotic treatment program and compounder for narcotic treatment program must maintain the following inventories and records of controlled substances:

- Inventories and records of controlled substances listed in Schedules I and II must be maintained separately from all of the records of the registrant; and

- Inventories and records of controlled substances listed in Schedules III, IV, and V must be maintained either separately from all other records of the registrant or in such form that the information required is readily retrievable from the ordinary business records of the registrant.

Inventory Requirements

Every required inventory and other records must be kept by the registrant and be available, for at least 2 years from the date of such inventory or records, for inspection and copying by authorized employees of the DEA.

Financial and shipping records (such as invoices and packing slips) may be kept at a central location (e.g. at the main office of a chain pharmacy), rather than at the registered location, if the registrant has notified the DEA of his intention to keep central records.

In order to keep centralized records, the following conditions must be met:

- Written notification must be submitted by registered or certified mail, return receipt requested, in triplicate, to the Special Agent in Charge of the DEA in the area in which the registrant is located. Unless the Special Agent in Charge informs the registrant that permission to keep central records is denied, the registrant may maintain central records commencing 14 days after receipt of his notification by the Special Agent in Charge.

- The notification must include:

  - The nature of the records to be kept centrally.

  - The exact location where the records will be kept.

  - The name, address, DEA registration number and type of DEA registration of the registrant whose records are being maintained centrally.

  - Whether central records will be maintained in a manual, or computer readable form.

- No executed order forms, prescriptions and/or inventories may be kept at the central location (they must be maintained at the registered location.

- If the records are kept on microfilm, computer media or in any form requiring special equipment to render the records easily readable, the registrant must provide access to such equipment with the records.

- The registrant must deliver all or any part of such records to the registered location or permit employees of DEA to inspect such records within two business days upon receipt of a written request from the DEA.

Each controlled substance inventory must contain a complete and accurate record of all controlled substances on hand on the date the inventory is taken, and must be maintained in written, typewritten, or printed form at the registered location. An inventory taken by use of an oral recording device must be promptly transcribed.

Controlled substances must be inventoried if they are in the possession of or under the control of the registrant. These include substances

- returned by a customer
- ordered by a customer but not yet invoiced
- stored in a warehouse on behalf of the registrant
- in the possession of employees of the registrant and intended for distribution as complimentary samples.

A separate inventory must be made for each registered location and each independent activity registered. In the event controlled substances in the possession or under the control of the registrant are stored at a location for which he/she is not registered, the substances must be included in the inventory of the registered location to which they are subject to control or to which the person possessing the substance is responsible.

The inventory may be taken either as of opening of business or as of the close of business on the inventory date and this must be indicated on the inventory.

Every registrant is required to take an inventory of all stocks of controlled substances on hand on the date he/she first engages in the manufacture, distribution, or dispensing of controlled substances. In the event a person commences business with no controlled substances on hand, he/she must record this fact as the initial inventory.

After the initial inventory is taken, the registrant must take a new inventory of all stocks of controlled substances on hand at least every two years. The biennial inventory may be taken on any date that is within two years of the previous biennial inventory date.

Note

A controlled substance inventory must be taken at least once every two years.

When the status of a noncontrolled substance is changed to that of a controlled substance, each registrant who possesses that substance must take an inventory of all stocks of the substance on hand. Thereafter, such substance must be included in each inventory made by the registrant.

When conducting a controlled substance inventory, the registrant must make an exact count of substances in sealed, unopened containers. For opened containers the following should be performed:

- If the substance is listed in Schedule I or II, make an exact count or measure of the contents.

- If the substance is listed in Schedule III, IV or V, make an estimated count or measure of the contents, unless the container holds more than 1,000 tablets or capsules in which case he/she must make an exact count of the contents.

Every registrant must maintain on a current basis a complete and accurate record of each controlled substance manufactured, imported, received, sold, delivered, exported, or otherwise disposed of by him/her. The records must be maintained in a dispensing log at the narcotic treatment program site. No registrant is required to maintain a perpetual inventory.

Each person registered or authorized to maintain and/or detoxify users of controlled substance, as part of a narcotic treatment program, must maintain records with the following information for each narcotic controlled substance:

- Name of substance
- Strength of substance
- Dosage form
- Date dispensed
- Adequate identification of patient (consumer)
- Amount consumed
- Amount and dosage form taken home by patient
- Dispenser's initials

All sites that compound a bulk narcotic solution from bulk narcotic powder to liquid for on-site use must keep a separate batch record of the compounding.

Records of identity, diagnosis, prognosis, or treatment of any patients, which are maintained in connection with the operation of a narcotic treatment program, must be confidential.

Extensive record keeping is required of individuals authorized to compound narcotic drugs for off-site use in a narcotic treatment program.

Section H

Treatment of Narcotic Dependence

The use of methadone as a way to wean narcotic-dependent individuals from opiates began with the passage of the Comprehensive Drug Abuse Prevention and Control Act of 1970. This approach to treatment has been very controversial because methadone itself is a controlled substance capable of being abused and has at times been diverted into illicit channels. The Narcotic Addict Treatment Act of 1974 provided for more stringent controls of methadone use and restricted its dispensing to practitioners who were registered with DEA and in compliance with the Drug Abuse Prevention and Control Act. In many cases, individual states have created their own legislation to control the use of methadone and similar drugs.

- The following is a synopsis of the most important elements of federal law as it applies to the treatment of narcotic dependence. Candidates should review these laws and regulations carefully, with particular emphasis on the role of the pharmacist and the specific use and control of methadone and levo-alpha-acetyl-methadol (LAAM).

Definitions

Detoxification treatment - dispensing of a narcotic drug in decreasing doses to an individual to alleviate adverse physiological or psychological effects incident to withdrawal from the continuous or sustained use of a narcotic drug and as a method of bringing the individual to a narcotic drug-free state within such period. There are two types of detoxification treatment: short-term detoxification treatment and long-term detoxification treatment.

- Short-term detoxification treatment is for a period not in excess of 30 days.
- Long-term detoxification treatment is for a period more than 30 days but not in excess of 180 days.

Maintenance Treatment - the dispensing of a narcotic drug, at relatively stable dosage levels, in the treatment of an individual for dependence on heroin or other morphine-like drug. There are two types of maintenance treatment: comprehensive maintenance treatment and interim maintenance treatment.

- Comprehensive maintenance treatment is maintenance treatment provided in conjunction with a comprehensive range of appropriate medical and rehabilitative services.

- Interim maintenance treatment is maintenance treatment provided in conjunction with appropriate medical services while a patient is awaiting transfer to comprehensive maintenance treatment.

Medical Director - is a physician, licensed to practice medicine in the jurisdiction in which the program is located. This individual assumes responsibility for the administration of all medical services performed by the narcotic treatment program, including ensuring that the program is in compliance with all federal, state, and local laws and regulations regarding the medical treatment of narcotic addiction with a narcotic drug.

Medication Unit - a facility established as part of, but geographically dispersed, (i.e., separate) from a narcotic treatment program from which licensed private practitioners and community pharmacists:

- are permitted to administer and dispense a narcotic drug, and
- are authorized to collect samples for drug testing or analysis for narcotic drugs

Narcotic Dependent - an individual who physiologically needs heroin or a morphine-like drug to prevent the onset of signs of withdrawal.

Narcotic Treatment Program - an organization (or a person, including a private physician) that administers or dispenses a narcotic drug to a narcotic addict for maintenance or detoxification treatment. It provides, when appropriate or necessary, a comprehensive range of medical and rehabilitative services, is approved by the state authority and the Food and Drug Administration, and that is registered with the DEA to use a narcotic drug for the treatment of narcotic addiction.

Program Sponsor - a person (or representative of an organization) who is responsible for the operation of a narcotic treatment program and who assumes responsibility for all its employees including any practitioners, agents, or other persons providing services at the program (including its medication units).

Services - includes medical evaluations, counseling, rehabilitative and other social programs (e.g., vocational and educational guidance, employment placement), which will help the patient become a productive member of society.

State Authority - is the agency designated by the Governor or other appropriate official to exercise the responsibility and authority within the State or Territory for governing the treatment of narcotic addiction with a narcotic drug.

Organizational Structure of Narcotic Treatment Programs

A narcotic treatment program may be an independent organization or part of a centralized organization. For example, if a centralized organizational structure consists of a primary facility and other outpatient facilities, all of which conduct initial evaluation of patients and administer or dispense medication, the primary facility and each outpatient facility are separate programs, even though some services (e.g., the same hospital or rehabilitative services) are shared.

The Program Sponsor is required to submit to the Food and Drug Administration and the State authority a description of the organizational structure of the program, the name of the persons responsible for the program, the address of the program, and the responsibilities of each facility or medication unit. The sources of funding for each program must be listed and the name and address of each governmental agency providing funding must be provided

Where two or more programs share a central administration (e.g., a city or state-wide organization), the person responsible for the organization (administrator or program sponsor) is required to be listed as the program sponsor for each separate participating program. An individual program must indicate its participation in the central organization at the time of its application. The administrator or sponsor may fulfill all record-keeping and reporting requirements for these programs, but each program must continue to receive separate approval.

One physician may assume primary medical responsibility for more than one program and be listed as medical director. If a physician assumes medical responsibility for more than one program, a statement documenting the feasibility of the arrangement must be attached to the application.

A public or nonprofit private narcotic treatment program may provide interim maintenance treatment only if the program also provides comprehensive maintenance treatment to which interim maintenance treatment patients may be transferred.

Program Approval

Before a narcotic treatment program may be lawfully operated, the program, whether an outpatient facility or a private practitioner, must submit the applications specified in this section simultaneously to the Food and Drug Administration and the state authority and must receive the approval of both.

Only program site(s) approved by federal, state, and local authorities may treat narcotic addicts with a narcotic drug. To obtain program approval, the applicant must demonstrate that he or she will have access to adequate physical facilities to provide all necessary services. A program must have ready access to a comprehensive range of medical and rehabilitative services so that the services may be provided when necessary. The name, address, and description of each hospital, institution, clinical laboratory, or other facility available to provide the necessary services are required to be included in the application submitted to the Food and Drug Administration and the state authority. The application is also required to include the name and address of each medication unit.

The following applications must be filed simultaneously with both the Food and Drug Administration and the state authority:

- Form FDA-2632 "Application for Approval of Use of Narcotic Drugs in a Treatment Program." This form, must be completed and signed by the program sponsor and submitted in duplicate to the Food and Drug Administration and the state authority.

- Form FDA-2633 ``Medical Responsibility Statement for Use of Narcotic Drugs in a Treatment Program." This form must be completed and signed by each licensed physician authorized to administer or dispense narcotic drugs and submitted in duplicate to the Food and Drug Administration and the state authority. The names of any other persons licensed by law to administer or dispense narcotic drugs working in the program must be listed even if they are not responsible for administering or dispensing the drug at the time the application is submitted.

No shipment of a narcotic drug may lawfully be made to any program that does not have current approval from the Food and Drug Administration. Within 60 days after receipt of the application from the program sponsor for approval, the Food and Drug Administration will notify the sponsor whether the application is approved or denied.

Before granting approval, the FDA must consult with the DEA (Department of Justice), to ascertain if the program is in compliance with Federal controlled substances laws. Each physical location within any program must be identified and listed in the approval application. At the time of application for approval, the program sponsor must indicate whether medication will be administered or dispensed at the facility. Before medication may be administered or dispensed at a location not previously approved for this purpose, the program is required to obtain approval from FDA and the state agency. However, no approval is necessary, but notification is required when a program deletes a facility in which medication is administered or dispensed. In that event, the program must notify the Food and Drug Administration and the state authority within three weeks of the deletion. Similarly, addition or deletion of facilities that provide services other than administering or dispensing medication is also permitted without approval, but notification must be made within three weeks to the Food and Drug Administration and the state authority about the addition and/or deletion.

State approval is not required for programs operated directly by the Veterans' Administration or any other department or agency of the United States. However, federal agencies operating narcotic treatment programs have agreed to cooperate voluntarily with State agencies by granting permission on an informal basis for designated state representatives to visit federal narcotic treatment programs and by furnishing a copy of federal reports to the state authority.

Services Provided by Treatment Programs

Each narcotic treatment program must provide medical and rehabilitative services and programs). These services should normally be made available at the primary facility, but the program sponsor may enter into a formal documented agreement with private or public agencies, organizations, or institutions for these services if they are available elsewhere. The program sponsor, in any event, must be able to document that medical and rehabilitative services are fully available to patients.

No prescribing, administering, or dispensing of a narcotic drug for the treatment of narcotic addiction may occur without prior approval by the Food and Drug Administration and the state authority, except if it a federal facility.

The following narcotic drugs have been approved for use in the treatment of narcotic addiction:

- methadone
- levo-alpha-acetyl-methadol (LAAM).

Medication Units

A program may establish a medication unit to facilitate the needs of patients who are stabilized on an optimal dosage level. To lawfully operate a medication unit, the program must, for each separate unit, obtain approval from the Food and Drug Administration, the Drug Enforcement Administration, and the state authority. If the Food and Drug

Administration revokes the primary program's approval, the approval for any medication unit associated with the program is automatically revoked. The Food and Drug Administration's revocation of the approval of a particular medication unit, will not, in and of itself, affect the approval of the primary program.

A medication unit must receive its supply of narcotic drugs directly from the stocks of the primary facility. Only persons permitted to administer or dispense the drug or security personnel licensed or otherwise authorized by state law to do so may deliver the drug to a medication unit.

The patient must be stabilized at his or her optimal dosage level before he or she may be referred to a medication unit. Since the medication unit does not provide a range of services, the program sponsor must determine that the patient to be referred is not in need of frequent counseling, rehabilitative, and other services that are only available at the primary program facility.

A medication unit is limited to administering or dispensing a narcotic drug and collecting samples for drug testing or analysis for narcotic drugs. If a private practitioner wishes to provide other services besides administering or dispensing a narcotic drug and collecting samples for drug testing or analysis for narcotic drugs, he or she must submit an application for separate approval.

After a patient is referred to a medication unit, the program sponsor retains continuing responsibility for the patient's care. The program sponsor must ensure that the patient receives needed medical and rehabilitative services at the primary facility.

An individual listed as program sponsor for a treatment program using a narcotic drug need not personally be a licensed practitioner but must employ a licensed physician for the position of medical director. Persons responsible for administering or dispensing the narcotic drug must be practitioners as defined by the CSA and licensed to practice by the state in which the program is to be established.

Admission to a Treatment Program

To be admitted to a treatment program an individual must:

- have a history of addiction and current physiologic dependence. A person may be admitted as a patient for a comprehensive maintenance program only if a program physician determines that the person is currently physiologically dependent upon a narcotic drug and became physiologically dependent at least one year before admission for comprehensive maintenance treatment.

- sign the "Consent to Treatment with an Approved Narcotic Drug" (Form FDA-2635). A parent, legal guardian, or responsible adult designated by the state may sign for patients under the age of 18.

A person who has resided in a penal or chronic care institution for 1 month or longer may be admitted to comprehensive maintenance treatment within 14 days before release or discharge, or within 6 months after release from such an institution without documented evidence to support findings of physiological dependence. However, the person must have been eligible for admission before he or she was incarcerated or institutionalized and, in the reasonable clinical judgment of a program physician, treatment is medically justified.

Treatment for Pregnant Patients

Pregnant patients, regardless of age, who have had a documented narcotic dependency in the past and who may return to narcotic dependency, with all its attendant dangers during pregnancy, may be placed on a comprehensive maintenance regimen. For such patients, evidence of current physiological dependence on narcotic drugs is not needed if a program physician certifies the pregnancy and, in his or her reasonable clinical judgment, finds treatment to be medically justified.

If a program cannot provide direct prenatal care for pregnant patients in treatment, the program must establish a system for informing the patients of the publicly or privately funded prenatal care opportunities available.

If a pregnant patient refuses direct treatment or appropriate referral for treatment, the treating program physician should consider using informed consent procedures (e.g., to have the patient acknowledge in writing that she had the opportunity for this treatment but refuses it.

Within 3 months after termination of pregnancy, the program physician must enter an evaluation of the patient's treatment state into her record and state whether she should remain in the comprehensive maintenance program or be detoxified.

Patients who are or become pregnant must not be started or continued on LAAM, except by the written order of a physician who determines this to be the best choice of therapy for that patient. Clinics providing treatment with LAAM must advise all patients of childbearing potential of the risks of LAAM and make a medical evaluation available to all patients who become pregnant while taking the drug. An initial pregnancy test must be performed for each prospective female patient of childbearing potential before admission to LAAM comprehensive maintenance treatment and monthly pregnancy tests performed thereafter on such female patients in LAAM comprehensive maintenance treatment.

Treatment of Minors

No person under 18 years of age may be admitted to a maintenance treatment program unless a parent, legal guardian, or responsible adult designated by the state authority (e.g., "emancipated minor" laws) completes and signs consent form, Form FDA-2635 "Consent to Treatment with an Approved Narcotic Drug." A person under 18 years of age may not be admitted to LAAM maintenance treatment.

Drug Testing

An initial drug-screening test or analysis must be completed for each prospective patient. At least eight additional random tests or analyses are performed on each patient during the first year in comprehensive maintenance treatment. In addition, at least quarterly random tests or analyses must be performed on each patient in comprehensive maintenance treatment for each subsequent year. A random test or analysis must be performed monthly on each patient who receives a 6-day supply of take-home medication.

When a sample is collected from each patient for such test or analysis, it must be done in a manner that minimizes opportunity for falsification. Each test or analysis must be analyzed for opiates, methadone, amphetamines, cocaine, and barbiturates. In addition, if any other drug or drugs have been determined by a program to be abused in that program's locality, or as otherwise indicated, each test or analysis must be analyzed for any of those drugs as well.

Test results may not be used as the sole criterion to force a patient out of treatment but may be used as a guide to change treatment approaches.

Authorized Dispensers of Narcotic Drugs

A narcotic drug may be administered or dispensed only by a practitioner licensed under the appropriate state law and registered under the appropriate state and federal laws to order narcotic drugs for patients, or by an agent of such a practitioner, supervised by and under the order of the practitioner. This agent is required to be a pharmacist, registered nurse, or licensed practical nurse or any other health care professional authorized by federal and state law to administer or dispense narcotic drugs. The licensed practitioner assumes responsibility for the amounts of narcotic drugs administered or dispensed and must record and countersign all changes in dosage schedule.

Note

Only a licensed physician, pharmacist, registered nurse, or licensed practical nurse may administer or dispense narcotics to patients as part of a narcotic treatment program. These health professionals must be employees of the program.

Methadone Use

Comprehensive Treatment

The person(s) responsible for the program must ensure that the initial dose of methadone does not exceed 30 milligrams and that the total dose for the first day does not exceed 40 milligrams, unless the program medical director documents in the patient's record that 40 milligrams did not suppress opiate abstinence symptoms. A licensed physician must assume responsibility for the amount of the narcotic drug administered or dispensed and must record, date, and sign in each patient's record each change in the dosage schedule. The administering licensed physician must ensure that a daily dose greater than 100 milligrams is justified in the patient's record.

Methadone may be administered or dispensed in oral form only when used in a treatment program. Hospitalized patients under care for a medical or surgical condition are permitted to receive methadone in parenteral form when the attending physician judges it advisable. Although tablet, syrup concentrate, or other formulations may be distributed to the program, all oral medication must be administered or dispensed in a liquid formulation. The oral dosage form must be formulated in such a way as to reduce its potential for parenteral abuse.

Take-home medication is required to be labeled with the treatment center's name, address, and telephone number and must be packaged in a child-resistant container to reduce the chances of accidental ingestion. Take-home medication may be given only to a patient who, in the reasonable clinical judgment of the program physician, is responsible in handling narcotic drugs. Before the program physician reduces the frequency of a patient's clinical visits, she or he or a designated staff member must record the rationale for the decision in the patient's clinical record. The program physician must consider the following in determining whether, in his or her reasonable clinical judgment, a patient is responsible in handling narcotic drugs:

- Absence of recent abuse of drugs (narcotic or non-narcotic), including alcohol
- Regularity of clinic attendance
- Absence of serious behavioral problems at the clinic
- Absence of known recent criminal activity (e.g., drug dealing)
- Stability of the patient's home environment and social relationships
- Length of time in comprehensive maintenance treatment
- Assurance that take-home medication can be safely stored within the patient's home
- Whether the rehabilitative benefit to the patient derived from decreasing the frequency of clinic attendance outweighs the potential risks of diversion.

Patients must come to the clinic for observation daily or at least 6 days a week. If, in the reasonable clinical judgment of the program physician, a patient demonstrates that he or she has satisfactorily adhered to program rules for at least 3 months, has made substantial progress in rehabilitation and responsibility in handling narcotic drugs, and would improve his or her rehabilitative progress by decreasing the frequency of attendance at the clinic for observation, the patient may be permitted to reduce his or her attendance at the clinic for observation to three times weekly. The patient may not receive more than a 2-day take-home supply of medication.

If, in the reasonable clinical judgment of the program physician, a patient demonstrates that he or she has satisfactorily adhered to program rules for at least two years from his or her entrance into the program, and meets the guidelines above, the patient may be permitted to reduce his or her clinic attendance at the clinic for observation to twice weekly. Such a patient may receive no more than a 3-day take-home supply of medication.

If, in the reasonable clinical judgment of the program physician, a patient demonstrates that he or she has satisfactorily adhered to program rules for at least three consecutive years from his or her entrance into the comprehensive maintenance treatment program, and meets the guidelines above, the patient may be permitted to reduce clinic attendance for observation to once weekly, provided that the following additional criteria are met:

- The program physician has written into the patient's record an evaluation that the patient is responsible in handling narcotic drugs.

- The patient is employed (or actively seeking employment), attends school, is a homemaker, or is considered unemployable for mental or physical reasons by a program physician.

- The patient is not known to have abused drugs including alcohol in the last year

- The patient is not known to have engaged in criminal activity (e.g., drug dealing), in the last year.

A patient permitted to reduce clinic attendance for observation to once weekly may not receive more than a 6-day take-home supply of medication.

If a patient, after receiving a supply of take-home medication, is inexcusably absent from or misses a scheduled appointment with a treatment program without authorization from the program staff, the program physician shall increase the frequency of the patient's clinic attendance for drug ingestion under observation. For such a patient, the program physician must not reduce the frequency of the patient's clinic attendance for drug ingestion under observation until she or he has had at least three consecutive monthly tests or analyses that are neither positive for morphine-like drugs (except from the narcotic drug administered or dispensed by the program) or other drugs of abuse, nor negative for the narcotic drug administered or dispensed by the program, and until she or he is again determined by a program physician to be responsible in handling narcotic drugs.

If a patient, after receiving a 6-day supply of take-home medication, has a test or analysis which is confirmed to be positive for morphine-like drugs (except for the narcotic drug administered or dispensed by the program) or other drugs of abuse, or negative for the narcotic drug administered or dispensed by the program, the program physician must place the patient on probation for 3 months. If, during this probation, the patient has a test or analysis either positive for morphine-like drugs (except for the narcotic drug administered or dispensed by the program) or other drugs of abuse, or negative for the narcotic drug administered or dispensed by the program, the program physician must increase the frequency of the patient's clinic attendance for observation to at least twice weekly. Such a patient may receive no more than a three-day take-home supply of medication until she or he has had at least three consecutive monthly tests or analyses which are neither positive for morphine-like drugs (except for the narcotic drug administered or dispensed by the program) or other drugs of abuse, nor negative for the narcotic drug administered or dispensed by the program, and the program physician again determines that the patient is responsible in handling narcotic drugs.

Each patient whose daily dose is above 100 milligrams is required to be under observation while ingesting the drug at least 6 days per week irrespective of the length of time in treatment, unless the program has received prior approval from the Food and Drug Administration with the concurrence of the state authority. An exception to this rule may be granted to patients with physical disabilities, illness, family crisis, or other hardship if they are deemed to be responsible in handling narcotic drugs. In any event, a patient may not be given more than a two-week supply of narcotic drugs at one time.

Short-term Detoxification Treatment

For short-term detoxification from narcotic drugs, the narcotic drug must be administered by the program physician or by an authorized agent of the physician, supervised by and under the order of the physician. The narcotic drug is required to be administered daily, under close observation, in reducing dosages over a period not to exceed 30 days. All requirements for comprehensive maintenance treatment apply to short-term detoxification treatment with the following exceptions:

- Take-home medication is not allowed during short-term detoxification.
- A history of 1-year physiologic dependence is not required for admission to short-term detoxification.

- Patients who have been determined by the program physician to be currently physiologically narcotic dependent may be placed in short-term detoxification treatment, regardless of age.

- No test or analysis is required except for the initial drug screening test or analysis.

- The initial treatment plan and periodic treatment plan evaluation required for comprehensive maintenance patients are not necessary for short-term detoxification patients. However, a primary counselor must be assigned by the program to monitor a patient's progress toward the goal of short-term detoxification and possible drug-free treatment referral

- A patient is required to wait at least seven days between concluding a short-term detoxification treatment episode and beginning another. Before a short-term detoxification attempt is repeated, the program physician must document in the patient's record that the patient continues to be, or is again, physiologically dependent on narcotics.

- Short-term detoxification treatment is not recommended for a pregnant patient.

Long-term Detoxification Treatment

For long-term detoxification from narcotic drugs, the narcotic drug must be administered by the program physician or by an authorized agent of the physician, supervised by and under the order of the physician. The narcotic drug is required to be administered on a regimen designed to reach a drug-free state and to make progress in rehabilitation in 180 days or less.

Unlike comprehensive treatment

- long-term detoxification treatment requires that the patient be under observation while ingesting the drug daily or at least six days a week, for the duration of the long-term detoxification treatment

- a history of 1-year physiologic dependence is not required for admission to long-term detoxification. The program physician must document in the patient's record that short-term detoxification is not a sufficiently long enough treatment course to provide the patient with the additional program services he or she deems necessary for the patient's rehabilitation. The program physician must document this information in the patient's record before long-term detoxification may begin.

- Patients who have been determined by the program physician to be currently physiologically dependent on narcotics may be placed in long-term detoxification treatment, regardless of age.

- An initial drug screening test or analysis is required for each patient. And at least one additional random test or analysis must be performed monthly on each patient during long-term detoxification.

- The initial treatment plan and periodic treatment plan evaluation required for comprehensive maintenance patients are also required for long-term detoxification patients, except that the required periodic treatment plan evaluation is required to occur monthly. A patient is required to wait at least seven days between concluding a long-term treatment episode and beginning another. Before a long-term detoxification attempt is repeated, the program physician must document in the patient's record that the patient continues to be or is again physiologically dependent on narcotic drugs. Long-term detoxification is not recommended for a pregnant patient.

Drug Dispensing

The person(s) responsible for a program must ensure that accurate records traceable to specific patients are maintained showing dates, quantity, and batch or code marks of the drug dispensed. These records must be retained for a period of three years from the date of dispensing.

Adequate security is required to be maintained over drug stocks, over the manner in which it is administered or dispensed, over the manner in which it is distributed to medication units, and over the manner in which it is stored to guard against theft and diversion of the drug. The program is required to meet the security standards for the distribution and storage of controlled substances as required by CSA.

Hospitalized Patients

For hospitalized patients, the drug may be administered or dispensed in either oral or parenteral form. For hospitalized patients, the use of a narcotic drug for narcotic addict treatment may be administered or dispensed only for detoxification treatment. If a narcotic drug is administered for treatment of narcotic dependence for more than 180 days, the procedure is no longer considered detoxification but is, rather, considered maintenance treatment.

Only approved narcotic treatment programs may undertake maintenance treatment. This does not preclude the maintenance treatment of a patient who is hospitalized for treatment of medical conditions other than addiction and who requires temporary maintenance treatment during the critical period of his or her stay or whose enrollment in a program which has approval for maintenance treatment using narcotic drugs has been verified.

Hospitals must submit to the Food and Drug Administration and the state authority the name of the individual (e.g., pharmacist) responsible for receiving and securing supplies of narcotic drugs for the treatment of narcotic addicts. The individual responsible for supplies must ensure that the only persons who receive supplies of narcotic drugs are those who are authorized to do so by federal or state law.

Application for a hospital pharmacy to provide narcotic drugs for detoxification treatment must be submitted to the Food and Drug Administration and the state authority. Approval from both is required.

Before a hospital pharmacy may lawfully receive shipments of narcotic drugs for detoxification treatment, a responsible official must complete, sign, and file in duplicate with the FDA and the state authority Form FDA-2636, "Hospital Request for Methadone Detoxification Treatment". The pharmacy must also have received from the FDA a notice that the request has been approved.

Use of LAAM in Maintenance Programs

After a patient's tolerance to LAAM is established, LAAM must be administered no more frequently than every other day. The dosage of LAAM must be individualized at doses, frequencies, and under conditions of usage described in as follows:

- The persons responsible for the program must ensure that the initial dose of LAAM to a patient whose tolerance for the drug is unknown does not exceed 40 milligrams.

- The persons responsible for the program must ensure that the initial dose of LAAM for a previously stabilized methadone maintenance patient is less than or equal to 1.3 times the patient's daily methadone dose, not to exceed 120 milligrams.

A licensed physician must assume responsibility for the amount of the narcotic drug administered or dispensed and must record, date, and sign or countersign in each patient's record each change in dosage schedule.

The administering licensed physician must ensure that a single dose of LAAM greater than 140 milligrams is justified in the patient's record.

LAAM may be administered in oral form when used in a maintenance treatment program. Hospitalized patients under care for a medical or surgical condition are permitted to receive LAAM in oral form when the attending physician judges it advisable. Although syrup concentrate or other formulations may be distributed to the program, all oral medication must be administered in a liquid formulation.

Clinics that administer both LAAM and methadone must take appropriate measures, including contrasting color and taste, to ensure that dosage forms of LAAM and methadone are easily distinguished.

Take-home doses of LAAM are not permitted. A patient who is eligible for one or more take-home doses of methadone and who is unable to conform to the applicable mandatory LAAM dosing schedule because of exceptional circumstances such as illness, personal or family crises, travel, or other hardship, or official state holidays, may be temporarily transferred to methadone.

Take-home doses of methadone for a patient eligible for a planned temporary discontinuation of treatment with LAAM must be individualized at doses, frequencies, and under conditions of usage described in the approved labeling and the applicable provisions for take-home methadone medication.

Section I

Nonprescription Drugs

Labeling Requirements

Over-the-counter (OTC) or nonprescription status is granted to drugs and drug products that have been shown to be safe for use without a physician's supervision, are for conditions suitable for self-diagnosis, and have adequate written directions for self-use. Of major importance with OTC products is appropriate labeling, which is easily understood by the general public.

Federal law requires manufacturers to use a "seven-point" label on nonprescription products. Included on the label must be:

- name of the product
- name and address of the manufacturer, packer, or distributor
- net contents of the package
- established name of all active ingredients and certain inactive ingredients
- name of any habit-forming drug present
- cautions and warnings needed to protect the consumer
- adequate directions for use

If any of the above information is missing, the nonprescription product is considered misbranded.

Other required information on nonprescription product labeling may include:

- statement of the intended use of the drug (e.g. "for motion sickness")

- dosage range appropriate for different ages

- how often the OTC may be safely taken

- route or method of administration

- other factors that may affect the efficacy of the drug (example: "take before meals" or "take one hour before bedtime")

In March 1999 the FDA published new OTC regulations. The stated objective of the new legislation was to allow consumers to better understand OTC information. The law provides that labels of nonprescription drug products must present "Drug Facts" in a standard order (similar to the "nutrition facts" on food products). The order of presentation recommended is:

- active ingredients
- purpose
- uses
- warnings
- directions
- other information
- inactive ingredients

Figure 2 is an example of this new "Drug Facts" section. The legislation also provides that the warnings section of nonprescription labels include the statement "Ask your doctor or pharmacist about food or drug interactions". In addition, the simplified standard language on OTC labels will include the term "uses", not "indications". Use of the terms "precautions" and "contraindications" will be eliminated.

Drug Facts

Active ingredient (in each tablet) — ***Purpose***

Chlorpheniramine maleate 2 mg .... Antihistamine

Uses temporarily relieves these symptoms due to hay fever or other upper respiratory allergies: ■ sneezing ■ runny nose ■ itchy, watery eyes ■ itchy throat

Warnings

Ask a doctor before use if you have
■ glaucoma ■ a breathing problem such as emphysema or chronic bronchitis
■ trouble urinating due to an enlarged prostate gland

Ask a doctor or pharmacist before use if you are taking tranquilizers or sedatives

When using this product
■ you may get drowsy ■ avoid alcoholic drinks
■ alcohol, sedatives, and tranquilizers may increase drowsiness
■ be careful when driving a motor vehicle or operating machinery
■ excitability may occur, especially in children

If pregnant or breast-feeding, ask a health professional before use.
Keep out of reach of children. In case of overdose, get medical help or contact a Poison Control Center right away.

Directions

adults and children 12 years and over	take 2 tablets every 4 to 6 hours; not more than 12 tablets in 24 hours
children 6 years to under 12 years	take 1 tablet every 4 to 6 hours; not more than 6 tablets in 24 hours
children under 6 years	ask a doctor

Other information ■ store at 20–25° C (68–77° F) ■ protect from excessive moisture

Inactive ingredients D&C yellow no. 10, lactose, magnesium stearate, microcrystalline cellulose, pregelatinized starch

Figure 2 - Sample of the "Drug Facts" section of nonprescription drug product labels.

Tamper-resistant Packaging

After several instances of deliberate addition of poisons to commercial nonprescription drug packages on store shelves, the Tamper-resistant Packaging Act was passed. The intent of this regulation is to prevent the intentional contamination of over-the-counter products.

Some exemptions from the requirement include:

- Aerosol products
- Nonprescription products not accessible to the general public (such as those in hospitals and other institutions)
- Lozenges, and drugs in first aid kits

In November 1998, the act was clarified by using the term "Tamper-evident Packaging". It is intended to heighten consumer awareness of potential tampering, without implying that a particular package is difficult to open or it is "tamper-proof".

This legislation also requires that two-piece hard gelatin capsules must be sealed using a tamper-evident technology and that the packages containing the capsules have at least one tamper-evident feature.

Switching of Prescription Drugs to Nonprescription Status

Requests for the reclassification of a prescription-only drug to OTC status is accomplished by one of the following four mechanisms:

- If the drug is now a prescription drug, a full NDA (New Drug Application) requesting OTC status may be submitted to the FDA for its evaluation.

- The FDA may grant an exemption if it deems that prescription-only status is unnecessary for the protection of the public health.

- A supplement to the NDA may be filed. The FDA will then review the relative safety of the drug based upon previous marketing experience and lack of a history of adverse effects.

- The Nonprescription Drug Advisory Committee may recommend that a particular ingredient be converted to nonprescription status.

The Nonprescription Drug Advisory Committees were originally established to evaluate the numerous nonprescription products and individual ingredients currently on the market. The committees or panels, subdivided by therapeutic categories, submitted their conclusions to the FDA. As a result of their deliberations, OTC ingredients were classified into one of three categories.

- **Category I** Generally recognized as safe and effective (GRASE) for the claimed therapeutic indication

- **Category II** Not generally recognized as safe and effective or having unacceptable indications

- **Category III** Insufficient data available to permit final classification

Note

A potential question on either the NAPLEX® or the MPJE® may be to determine if the candidate is familiar with the status of a specific drug product. Drugs or drug products that were switched from Rx-only to nonprescription status within the past few years may be included. However, the exam will likely avoid including drug products whose status may change in the near future or those that are being presently evaluated for a change. It is unlikely that questions that ask for concentrations or strengths of prescription versus nonprescription products will be asked on the MPJE®.

Nonprescription Sale of Ipecac Syrup

While ipecac syrup contains the federal legend requiring dispensing only by prescription, there is one notable exception. A 30mL container of ipecac syrup may be sold as a nonprescription item. The intent of this exemption is to provide every household with an emetic for the immediate treatment of accidental poisoning.

To qualify for nonprescription sale

- Only 30mL containers of ipecac syrup may be sold.
- The bottle label must state in red letters: "For emergency use to cause vomiting in poisoning. Before using, call a physician, the Poison Control Center, or a hospital emergency room immediately for advice."

- The label should contain the warning: "Keep out of reach of children. Do not use in unconscious persons." "Do not use when strychnine, corrosives such as alkalies and strong acids, or petroleum distillates such as kerosene, gasoline, fuel, oil, paint thinner, or cleaning fluid have been ingested.

- The usual dosage of ipecac syrup in persons over one year of age is one tablespoonful (15mL).

Sample Questions

1. The maximum volume of Ipecac Syrup that may be sold without a prescription is:
   (A) 15 mL (B) 30 mL (C) 60 mL
   (D) 120 mL (E) > 120 mL

2. Under which of the following circumstances may Ipecac Syrup be sold without a prescription?
   I. For future use during accidental poisoning
   II. Only if the household does not have small children
   III. If the purchaser signs a pharmacy logbook
   (A) I only (B) III only (C) I & II only
   (D) II & III only (E) I, II, & III

3. The label of a bottle of Ipecac Syrup sold OTC for accidental poisoning must:
   I. state that the appropriate dose is the entire bottle followed by a full glass of water.
   II. provide the telephone number of a poison control center.
   III. must have its warnings printed in red ink.
   (A) I only (B) III only (C) I & II only
   (D) II & III only (E) I, II, & III

Answers: (1) B (2) A (3) B

Nonprescription Sale of Quinine

In 1998, the FDA classified nonprescription quinine products to be unsafe for the treatment and/or prevention of malaria. Previously the use of nonprescription quinine products for nocturnal leg cramps was discontinued because there was a lack of substantial evidence of its effectiveness as well as concerns about potential toxicity.

Section J

Dietary and Nutritional Products

Dietary Supplement Health Education Act (DSHEA)

This act exempts health foods, food supplements, and herbal products from the strict controls imposed by the FDA on prescription drugs and OTC drug products. Products included under DSHEA are vitamins, minerals, herbals, amino acids and related supplements. Provisions of this act include the following:

- Products may be marketed without their efficacy proven. This means that the FTC or FDA would have to challenge products after they have been introduced onto the market if there is evidence that they are ineffective for the advertised or labeled use.

- Products currently on the market do not have to be proven safe. It is the responsibility of the FDA to prove that a product is unsafe before it can be challenged. However the manufacturer must provide "reasonable" assurances that no ingredient in the product presents a significant or unreasonable risk of illness or injury.

- Product manufacturing processes do not have to meet FDA's GMPs. The FDA Good Manufacturing Practices are very detailed and strict. To manufacture drug products, every pharmaceutical manufacturer must submit specific details of their production facilities and describe how every product is processed. This is not required for dietary supplements, herbals, etc. However, this does not mean that these products can be made under unsanitary conditions. At the present time, dietary supplement and herbal manufacturers are deveoping GMP guidelines for these products.

Manufacturers are allowed to make structure/function claims on labels if the statements do not indicate that the product will diagnose, cure, treat, or prevent a disease. Some claims related to the product's ability to affect body structure or function are permitted if they are truthful and not misleading. For example, a claim that Saw Palmetto will "improve urinary flow" or that it is "for the prostate" is acceptable. A statement such as "will cure an enlarged prostate" is not acceptable. While the manufacturer must substantiate any product claims, they do NOT have to be reviewed or approved by FDA. The manufacturer must state this fact (i.e. that the FDA has not reviewed product claims) on the label.

Note

Since there is an ongoing dialogue between the FDA and manufacturers of the above products as to the interpretation of allowable claims, it is unlikely any specific questions about these products will appear on the MPJE® .

Official Status of Herbals

The USP/NF has developed monographs for some botanicals that appear to have therapeutic activity. For admission into the USP, the herb must have an FDA approved use or a USP DI Panel recognized use. At the present time, the active herbs have not been admitted to the USP but have been admitted to the NF when there are no significant safety concerns. The monographs describe the portions of plant used, its botanical characteristics, and appropriate assay procedures for ingredients. The monographs do not describe the therapeutic uses of the herb. Monographs are currently available for chamomile, cranberry liquid preparation, feverfew, garlic, ginger, ginkgo, milk thistle, St John's wort, saw palmetto, and valerian.

Sample Questions

Answer the following questions using the key of:

(A) I only (B) III only (C) I & II only
(D) II & III only (E) I, II, & III

1. Which of the following statements is (are) true?
   I. None of the herbals used in the US are recognized in the USP/NF.
   II. Commercial herbals may be categorized as nonprescription drug
   III. Commercial herbals are categorized as dietary supplements.

2. A pharmacist may sell herbals provided that:
   I. The patient is properly counseled with respect to their use.
   II. The consumer is cautioned to use the product for not more than two weeks.
   III. There are adequate directions on the package for patient use.

3. Upon formal request, to whom must the manufacturer of an herbal product submit data supporting the claims for the product?
   I. FDA or FTC
   II. pharmacists
   III. consumers

Answers: (1) B (2) B (3) A

Homeopathic Drug Products

The Federal Food, Drug and Cosmetic Act of 1938 recognized the Homeopathic Pharmacopoeia of the United States (HPUS) as an official compendium. Drug products that use an official name designation found in the HPUS must meet all of its compendial standards. Otherwise the drug product is misbranded or adulterated.

The basic elements of homeopathic medicine include individualized dosing of patients by homeopathic physicians, based upon a patient's symptoms. The dose of drug administered is usually extremely low; often dilutions of 1:1,000 or 1:1,000,000 are used with frequent drug administration. These drug products must meet the usual drug labeling requirements including ingredient names, amounts, and directions for use. While many of the drugs were originally labeled by their Latin name, it is now required that their English name be provided. Some of the drugs found in homeopathic formulas are also official in the USP/NF. In these situations, the drug must meet the stricter standards found in the USP/NF. If the drug product is intended for nonprescription use, its label must include appropriate warning statements, if needed.

While homeopathic drugs must be manufactured under GMP standards, they do not have to have an expiration date on the package.

Section K

Cosmetics

The legal distinction between cosmetics and drugs is muddled. Some cosmetics, such as fluoridated toothpaste, medicated mouthwash, or anti-dandruff shampoos are borderline products. The overriding factor in determining a product's status may not be its ingredients, but what claims are made for the product, especially on the label.

While cosmetic manufacturers do not have to meet the rigorous requirements of the FDA's good manufacturing practices (GMP's), they are still obligated to manufacture under sanitary conditions. Otherwise, their products may be classified as being adulterated. While the Federal Food, Drug, and Cosmetic Act of 1938 does not specifically state that cosmetics have to be tested for safety, any cosmetic that poses a safety problem to the general public will be considered as being misbranded. If an unapproved color additive is used in the formulation, the product will be classified as being adulterated.

Regulation of advertising and labeling of cosmetics basically falls under the jurisdiction of the Federal Trade Commission (FTC). On cosmetic product labels, ingredients must be listed in descending order of predominance. (that is why water may be listed as the first ingredient, while the "active ingredient" is listed further down in the ingredient list). Ingredients present in quantities of one percent or less may be listed at the bottom, in random order. The listed names must be the generic names established by the cosmetic industry, usually by the Cosmetic, Toiletry, and Fragrance Association (CTFA). Perfumes and flavoring oils may simply be listed by name. Coloring agents must be those accepted for cosmetic use. A minor exception to the above ingredient listing requirement are cosmetics used in professional settings such as by professional hairdressers (i.e. cosmetics not intended for retail sales).

Many cosmetic products, especially those intended for use in body cavities (e.g. mouthwashes and vaginal products) must be packaged in tamper-resistant packaging.

Section L

Miscellaneous Laws and Regulations

Alcohol Regulations

The Bureau of Alcohol, Tobacco and Firearms controls the sale of alcohol. Pharmacies may purchase 95% ethanol (190 proof grain alcohol) for routine compounding by using Form ATF-11. If a pharmacy is selling alcohol in the form of a beverage, it must obtain a retail liquor dealer's stamp. Institutions that have a need for greater volumes of alcohol may choose to purchase tax-free alcohol since it is much lower in cost (tax on regular alcohol purchases is very high). Such pharmacies must purchase alcohol by using Form ATF-1447.

The following are federal statutes that relate to the use of tax-free alcohol:

- Its use is limited to medicinal or scientific use, or in patient treatment.

- The alcohol can not be sold or loaned to other pharmacies or physician's offices.

- The alcohol, either by itself or as a component of other products, may not be sold to outpatients. An exception to this requirement permits nonprofit clinics to dispense medicines made with tax-free alcohol provided the client is not charged for the medication.

- Running, accurate inventories must be kept on all alcohol in stock.

- Containers of alcohol, usually supplied in 10 or 55 gallon drums, must be stored in a securely locked, fire-resistant storeroom.

How may a prescriber's order for an alcohol-containing beverage (e.g. brandy at bedtime) for an institutionalized client be handled? Either

- the institution may buy the alcohol-containing beverage, furnish it to the client, and then bill the patient.

- the hospital pharmacy may give the patient's relatives permission to bring alcohol in for the patient.

Other available forms of tax-exempt alcohol are the Specially Denatured Alcohols (SDAs). SDA's refers to specific formulas of grain alcohol that have been rendered unsuitable for use as a beverage by the addition of denaturants such as sucrose octaacetate, brucine, or butyl alcohol. There are a large number of formulas for SDAs, usually designated as SDA 40A, SDA 23H, etc. SDA are often used for pharmaceutical processing and in commercial products such as mouthwashes.

Americans with Disabilities Act (ADA)

The Federal Rehabilitation Act of 1973 prevents an employer from discriminating against a handicapped person who is otherwise qualified to perform the functions of a job. The Act applies only to those companies receiving federal assistance. The employee's handicap could be either mental or physical. The Americans with Disabilities Act (ADA) was passed in 1990 with an effective date in 1992. This act expands the original Rehabilitation Act by greatly increasing the number of individuals covered and by covering companies even if they are not receiving federal financial assistance. Any company employing 15 or more people is covered. In both acts, the term "disabled" is used since it has less of a negative connotation than the term "handicapped".

These acts provide civil rights protection to individuals with disabilities similar to those provided to individuals on the basis of race, color, sex, national origin, age, and religion. Among those covered under the ADA are individuals with epilepsy, paralysis, HIV infections, AIDS, mental retardation, and alcoholics. Those NOT protected are individuals who illegally use drugs. A key concept of both acts is that employers must make a “reasonable effort” to accommodate a disabled employee.

In addition to the elements of these laws specified above are the following:

- The employer must make reasonable accommodations for disabled individuals whether those individuals are employees or members of the general public. For the general public, "reasonable accommodations" include providing ramps leading into a building, providing elevator service to all floors of a building, and constructing restroom facilities that are accessible to disabled individuals.

- For an employee, "reasonable accommodations" might be a reduced-height workbench.

- An employer may not ask about disabilities during an employment interview, but may ask if the prospective employee has the ability to perform the work.

Note

A court has ruled that persons with HIV infections may not be discriminated against by either refusing them employment or by refusing to assign them to the usual daily functions of a pharmacist. This concept could be extended to pregnant female pharmacists who may wish to prepare chemotherapy drug admixtures. Obviously if they prefer NOT to work with potential mutagenic agents, their wishes should be followed.

- An employer may not require a prospective employee to undergo a medical examination before offering a position. However, the employer may require a medical examination as a condition of employment if this is a requirement for all new employees.

Note

Tests for illegal use of drugs are not considered to be medical examinations and may be required by an employer.

Sample Questions

1. The requirements of the ADA must be followed if what minimum number of employees is employed in a pharmacy
   (A) 2 (B) 10 (C) 15 (D) 50 (E) 100

2. Which of the following conditions may preclude a pharmacist from working in a hospital pharmacy?
   I. alcoholism
   II. HIV infection
   III. cocaine addiction
   (A) I only (B) III only (C) I & II only
   (D) II & III only (E) I, II, & III

3. An institutional pharmacy employer may NOT prevent pharmacists with which of the following conditions from working in a parenteral admixture room?
   I. chronic alcoholism
   II. HIV infection
   III. epilepsy
   (A) I only (B) III only (C) I & II only
   (D) II & III only (E) I, II, & III

4. The ADA protects an employee when an employer attempts to enforce:
   I. random locker-room searches for illegal drugs
   II. IQ tests
   III. weight reduction programs
   (A) I only (B) III only (C) I & II only
   (D) II & III only (E) I, II, & III

Answers: (1) C (2) B (3) E (4) D

Drug-free Workplace

According to the Federal Anti-Drug Abuse Act of 1988

- The unlawful possession of controlled substances by employees is prohibited in the work place.
- If an employee is convicted of criminal possession of drugs, he/she must inform the employer of the conviction within five days.
- Employers may take appropriate action.

Unfair Competition

It is unlikely that questions concerning the economical aspects of pharmacy will be asked on the MPJE®. However one should be aware of two major laws in this area.

Sherman Antitrust Act

The Sherman Antitrust Act prevents restraint of trade or the establishment of monopolies. Originally the Sherman Antitrust Act was intended to curtail the large monopolies that operated in the early 1900's. The concept of the Act is to prevent restraint of trade and/or the establishment of monopolies. Companies or groups may not have agreements, either formal or informal, among themselves, which would unreasonably restrain trade. For example, three independent pharmacies in a given area may not agree to a common drug mark-up of 40% or a professional fee of $4.24. These actions would probably be classified as price fixing. Other examples could be the distribution of suggested retail prices for certain prescription drugs by a pharmaceutical organization or the boycott by a group of pharmacies of a third party payer because of its low reimbursement rate. In addition, a group of pharmacies may not agree as a group to reject a third-party prescription plan nor can they collectively bargain for better reimbursement rates. However, a chain consisting of several pharmacies may do so.

Robinson-Patman Act

The intent of the Robinson-Patman Act is to prevent the hindering of competition. A seller is not allowed to practice price discrimination when dealing with similar purchasers. For example, the wholesale price for 100 x 1,000 tablet bottles may not favor one pharmacy over another. Likewise, this issue arises when individual states allow hospitals to dispense prescriptions to walk-in clients if the hospital has a community pharmacy permit. In this case, however, the price of the prescription may not be based upon the special, reduced price that the hospital received from the pharmaceutical manufacturer. Nor can the hospital sell drugs or medical devices to affiliated groups such as a home health care business at the special, reduced price.

Hospitals and similar institutions do have the right to extend their special prices to employees, inpatients, emergency room patients, etc. This is known as "own use". Institutions are not permitted to provide prescription refills for former patients unless the take-home drugs are intended as continued care or supplementing treatment administered in the hospital. For example, continuing a treatment with parenteral antibiotics.

While physicians on the hospital staff may be supplied with drugs for personal use, drugs cannot be sold to physicians for use in their private practice especially if they are to be sold to patients."

Section M

Sample Questions

1. The organization responsible for overseeing the selection of a nonproprietary name for a new drug is the:
(A) FDA (B) FTC (C) USAN
(D) USP/NF (E) APhA

2. Which of the following are examples of Schedule I substances?
I. Lysergic acid diethylamide
II. Mescaline
III. Peyote
(A) I only (B) III only (C) I & II only
(D) II & III only (E) I, II, & III

3. Pharmacists may transfer prescription information on a one-time basis for the purpose of refill dispensing for which of the following drug products?
I. Lomotil tablets
II. Dalmane capsules
III. Tylenol w/codeine capsules
(A) I only (B) III only (C) I & II only
(D) II & III only (E) I, II, & III

4. Which one of the following organizations is directly responsible for Medicare programs?
   (A) FDA (B) HCFA (C) HMO
   (D) JCAHO (E) AARP

5. A product that contains 60 mg of codeine and 325 mg of acetaminophen is most likely to be classified as
   (A) Schedule II (B) Schedule III (C) Schedule IV
   (D) ScheduleV (E) Noncontrolled

6. A new drug product is given the name " felorazepam". It is likely to be classified as
   (A) Schedule II (B) Schedule III (C) Schedule IV
   (D) ScheduleV (E) Noncontrolled

7. Which of the following barbiturates is classified in controlled substance category IV?
   I. Amobarbital
   II. Pentobarbital
   III. Phenobarbital
   (A) I only (B) III only (C) I & II only
   (D) II & III only (E) I, II, & III

8. A new cough syrup contains 15 mg of codeine phosphate and 100 mg of guaifenesin in each 10 mL dose. A 4 fluid ounce container of this product would likely be classified as
   (A) Schedule II (B) Schedule III (C) Schedule IV
   (D) ScheduleV (E) Noncontrolled

9. How may a physician obtain cocaine HCl powder for use as a local anesthetic in his office?
   I. He may write a prescription for the drug and write "for office use" on its face.
   II. He may write an order for the drug in an institutional setting and label it "for office use"
   III. He may order it directly from a supplier using DEA Form 222.
   (A) I only (B) III only (C) I & II only
   (D) II & III only (E) I, II, & III

10. Proposed regulations from the FDA are first published in the:
(A) Congressional Record (B) Federal Register
(C) New York Times and Wall Street Journal
(D) USP/NF (E) Supplements of the USP/NF

11. A physician telephones a pharmacy and prescribes 40 Percodan tablets, 1 TID. Which of the following is/are true?
I. It may only be dispensed in an emergency.
II. A written "cover" prescription must be received before the pharmacist may dispense the medication.
III. Not more than a 7-day supply may be prescribed orally.
(A) I only (B) III only (C) I & II only
(D) II & III only (E) I, II, & III

12. A pharmacist may issue a Power of Attorney to an individual in order to permit the individual to
I. fill controlled substance prescriptions.
II. conduct a narcotic treatment facility.
III. complete DEA Form 222 orders.
(A) I only (B) III only (C) I & II only
(D) II & III only (E) I, II, & III

13. A pharmacist who fills an oral morphine sulfate prescription in an emergency does not receive a "cover" prescription from the prescriber. The pharmacist must
I. notify the regional DEA office.
II. notify the state board of medicine.
III. call the patient and request that he/she obtain a written prescription to cover the oral order.
(A) I only (B) III only (C) I & II only
(D) II & III only (E) I, II, & III

14. A physician wishes to prescribe a schedule II controlled substance for a patient residing in a hospice. How may the prescription be conveyed to a pharmacy?
    I. As a written prescription
    II. By fax
    III. By e-mail
    (A) I only (B) III only (C) I & II only
    (D) II & III only (E) I, II, & III

15. Under which of the following conditions may a pharmaceutical sales representative distribute samples of a prescription drug product?
    I. Upon written request from a community pharmacy
    II. Upon written request from a hospital pharmacy
    III. Upon written request from a physician
    (A) I only (B) III only (C) I & II only
    (D) II & III only (E) I, II, & III

16. Benzadrex Inhalers are an example of a product classified as
    (A) Schedule II (B) Schedule III (C) Schedule IV
    (D) ScheduleV (E) Noncontrolled

17. The expiration date on a commercial pharmaceutical product is July 2004. The actual date that this product will be considered expired will be after:
    (A) June 30th (B) July 1st (C) July 15th
    (D) July 31st (E) August 1st

18. A patient presents a prescription for sixty Empirin w/codeine tablets No.4 to his local pharmacy and indicates that he would only like to get 30 of the tablets now and will return for the other 30 in a week if the medication agrees with him. The pharmacist should
    (A) call the prescriber to get permission to dispense 30.
    (B) dispense 30 tablets as requested by the patient.

(C) advise the patient that the full 60 tablets must be supplied at one time.
(D) fill the prescription as requested by the patient but advise the patient that the balance must be picked up within 72 hours.
(E) dispense 30 tablets of Empirin w/codeine No. 2 tablets.

19. Which of the following is/are true regarding the sale of codeine-containing schedule V cough medicine without a prescription?
I. Only a pharmacist may dispense the product to the consumer.
II. A non-pharmacist may "ring-up" the sale and collect payment for the product.
III. Not more than 120 mL or 24 dosage units of this product may be sold to the same purchaser in any 7-day period.
(A) I only (B) III only (C) I & II only
(D) II & III only (E) I, II, & III

20. A pharmacist who does not receive a registration renewal form from DEA within 45 days before the expiration of his/her registration must notify
I. his/her state's board of pharmacy
II. the regional FDA office
III. the DEA in writing and request renewal forms
(A) I only (B) III only (C) I & II only
(D) II & III only (E) I, II, & III

21. Which of the following reference book(s) is(are) legal documents recognized by the federal government?
I. *Remington's Pharmaceutical Sciences*
II. *Homeopathic Pharmacopeia of the U.S.*
III. *USP/NF*
(A) I only (B) III only (C) I & II only
(D) II & III only (E) I, II, & III

22. The Consumer Product Safety Commission is responsible for which one of the following?
    (A) Federal Food Drug, and Cosmetic Act
    (B) DSHEA
    (C) Prescription drug to OTC status
    (D) Poison Prevention Packaging Act
    (E) Good Manufacturing Practices

23. Which of the following sublingual tablets do NOT have to be dispensed in child-resistant containers?
    I. Nitroglycerin
    II. Nitrostat
    III. Isordil
    (A) I only (B) III only (C) I & II only
    (D) II & III only (E) I, II, & III

24. Which of the following drug products may be purchased by a pharmacy WITHOUT the use of a DEA Form 222?
    I. Lorcet Tablets
    II. Stadol
    III. Mepergan Injection
    (A) I only (B) III only (C) I & II only
    (D) II & III only (E) I, II, & III

25. Which of the following products are exempt from the FDA regulations concerning expiration dating?
    I. USP/NF drug products
    II. dietary supplements
    III. vitamins
    (A) I only (B) III only (C) I & II only
    (D) II & III only (E) I, II, & III

26. Guidelines for determining an expiration date for repackaging of a drug product by a pharmacy includes:
    I. not more than the expiration date on the original package
    II. not more than one year from the date of packaging
    III. one-half of the time remaining on the original package

(A) I only (B) III only (C) I & II only
(D) II & III only (E) I, II, & III

27. A physician who is a resident in a hospital and does not have a DEA registration number
    (A) may not prescribe controlled substances.
    (B) may only prescribe controlled substances for outpatients.
    (C) may prescribe controlled substances using the hospital DEA number plus an assigned suffix.
    (D) may prescribe controlled substances only in Schedule III-V
    (E) May prescribe only for inpatients

28. If a specific lot of a pharmaceutical company's tablets fails to meet the expected expiration dating, the lot may be considered to be:
    (A) adulterated
    (B) unstable
    (C) misbranded
    (D) a class III recall
    (E) a felony

29. The federal act that specifically limits the reimportation of drug products that were previously exported by a pharmaceutical manufacturer is the:
    (A) FD & C Act of 1938
    (B) Durham-Humphrey Act
    (C) Prescription Drug Marketing Act of 1987
    (D) DSHEA
    (E) Kefauver-Harris Amendment of 1962

30. A pharmacist may fill prescriptions for and mail which of the following drugs through the US Postal Service?
    I. Schedule II non-narcotics
    II. Benzodiazepines
    III. Schedule II narcotics

    (A) I only (B) III only (C) I & II only
    (D) II & III only (E) I, II, & III

31. Which of the following actions are appropriate when mailing a narcotic drug filled using a valid prescription?
    I. Package the drug container in a plain paper outer wrapping
    II. Place the warning: "Narcotic, do not open while in transit" on the outer wrapping
    III. Place a fictitious return address on the outer wrapping.
    (A) I only (B) III only (C) I & II only
    (D) II & III only (E) I, II, & III

32. Labels on cosmetic packages must have ingredients listed:
    (A) in descending order of concentration
    (B) ascending order of concentration
    (C) alphabetically
    (D) any random order
    (E) with the most active listed first

33. Samples of prescription drugs received from pharmaceutical companies may be
    (A) sold through community pharmacies
    (B) dispensed from a hospital pharmacy for inpatients
    (C) dispensed from a hospital to outpatients
    (D) given to patients by a prescriber
    (E) traded to another pharmacy for other drugs

34. Which of the following actions is (are) permissible under the FDA rules for prescription compounding by pharmacies?
    I. advertising to dermatologists that the pharmacy can compound topical antifungal ointments
    II. send brochures to nurse practitioners that the pharmacy compounds topical lotions for psoriasis
    III. Inform an allergist that the pharmacy can economically compound 50 mg diphenhydramine capsules
    (A) I only (B) III only (C) I & II only
    (D) II & III only (E) I, II, & III

35. Which of the following controlled drugs may a pharmacist mail through the US Postal Service?
    I. Schedule II's
    II. Schedule III's
    III. Schedule IV's
    (A) I only (B) III only (C) I & II only
    (D) II & III only (E) I, II, & III

36. A community pharmacy develops and prepares batches of 5,000 sustained release capsules similar to a commercially available product but at a lower price. The pharmacy may be cited for this activity based upon:
    I. The capsule formula may be considered a new drug
    II. The preparation of 5,000 capsules may be considered manufacturing.
    III. The failure to following GMPs.
    (A) I only (B) III only (C) I & II only
    (D) II & III only (E) I, II, & III

37. Which of the following would be violations of the Sherman Antitrust Act with respect to the two independent pharmacies X and Y?
    I. Pharmacy X decides to discontinue the selling of wheelchairs.
    II. Pharmacy X agrees to sell only electric wheelchairs if pharmacy Y sells only conventional wheelchairs.
    III. Pharmacies X and Y agree to rent wheelchairs at not less than $60.00 a month.
    (A) I only (B) III only (C) I & II only
    (D) II & III only (E) I, II & III

38. A patient presents a prescription for MS Contin tablets 30mg tablets # 60 to his local pharmacy and indicates that he would only like to get 30 of the tablets now and will return for the other 30 in a week if the medication agrees with him. The pharmacist should

(A) call the prescriber to get permission to dispense 30.
(B) dispense 30 tablets as requested by the patient.
(C) advise the patient that the full 60 tablets must be supplied at one time.
(D) fill the prescription as requested by the patient but advise the patient that the balance must be picked up within 72 hours.
(E) dispense 30 tablets of the 60 mg strength of MS Contin.

39. Which dosage forms of secobarbital must be ordered using a DEA Form 222?
I. Capsule
II. Injectable
III. Suppository
(A) I only (B) III only (C) I & II only
(D) II & III only (E) I, II, & III

40. Davis Labs is the first to place a new drug product on the market. This product would be described in the Orange Book as:
I. a reference drug product
II. B rated
III. AB rated
(A) I only (B) III only (C) I & II only
(D) II & III only (E) I, II, & III

41. Major objectives for developing a formulary include:
I. reduce drug inventory
II. allow therapeutic substitution
III. give prescribers a greater latitude of drug selection
(A) I only (B) III only (C) I & II only
(D) II & III only (E) I, II, & III

42. Which of the following protocols must a hospital pharmacy follow in order to possess pharmaceutical manufacturer's drug samples?
I. The hospital must be registered as a drug wholesaler.

II. The hospital must store the samples separate from the regular stock.
III. A licensed practitioner must have requested the samples from the company.
(A) I only (B) III only (C) I and II only
(D) II and III only (E) I, II, and III

43. Which of the following volumes of the USP/DI contains significant information concerning the bio-equivalence of drug products?
I. Volume I
II. Volume II
III. Volume III
(A) I only (B) III only (C) I & II only
(D) II & III only (E) I, II, & III

44. The major objective of the Orange Book is to compare drug products that are
I. multisourced
II. most economical
III. different dosage forms
(A) I only (B) III only (C) I & II only
(D) II & III only (E) I, II, & III

45. Which of the following was the first to require that pharmaceutical manufacturers prove the safety of prescription drugs before marketing?
(A) Durham-Humphrey Amendment (1951)
(B) F D & C Act of 1938
(C) Kefauver-Harris Amendment of 1962
(D) Prescription Drug Marketing Act of 1987
(E) Pure Food and Drug Act of 1906

46. Which of the following designations indicate that drug products of the same strength and dosage form may be interchangeable?
I. BC
II. AB
III. A

(A) I only (B) III only (C) I & II only
(D) II & III only (E) I, II, & III

47. The Orange Book uses the symbol "+", in a series of similar drug products to indicate:
(A) the drug product has not been assessed
(B) there is no bioequivalence problem
(C) the drug product that is preferred by most pharmacists for substitution
(D) indicates the least expensive drug product
(E) the product used as reference standard

48. Drug products with which of the following codes may be substituted for one another?
I. A
II. AB
III. B
(A) I only (B) III only C) I & II only
(D) II & III only (E) I, II, & III

Questions 49 - 57. Answer the next series of questions based ONLY upon the data presented in Figures A-C adapted from the Orange Book.

49. A prescription is written for Coumadin tablets 5 mg with an indication that substitution is desired. Which of the following manufacturers have suitable products? (see Figure A)
I. Dupont Merck
II. Invamed
III. Barr
(A) I only (B) III only (C) I & II only
(D) II & III only (E) I, II, & III

50. A prescription is written for warfarin tablets 2 mg with an indication that substitution is desired. Which of the following manufacturers have suitable products? (See Figure A)

I. Dupont Merck
II. Invamed
III. Barr

(A) I only (B) III only (C) I & II only
(D) II & III only (E) I, II, & III

WARFARIN SODIUM

TABLET; ORAL

COUMADIN

AB +	**DUPONT MERCK**	**1 mg**
AB +		**2 mg**
AB +		**5 mg**
AB +		**10 mg**

WARFARIN SODIUM

AB	**BARR**	**2 mg**
AB		**5 mg**
AB		**10 mg**
AB	**INVAMED**	**1 mg**
AB		**2 mg**
AB		**10 mg**

Figure A

51. In order to be considered bioequivalent with Dupont's Coumadin tablets, Barr's warfarin sodium tablets must have the same (See Figure A):
    I. color
    II. excipients
    III. drug level
    (A) I only (B) III only (C) I & II only
    (D) II & III only (E) I, II, & III

	NITROGLYCERIN	
	Film, Extended Release; Transdermal	
	NITRODUR	
AB1	**KEY**	**0.1 mg/hr**
AB1		**0.2 mg/hr**
AB1		**0.4 mg/hr**
AB1		**0.6 mg/hr**
AB1		**0.8 mg/hr**
	MINITRAN	
AB1	**3M**	**0.1 mg/hr**
AB1		**0.2 mg/hr**
AB1		**0.4 mg/hr**
AB1		**0.6 mg/hr**
	TRANSDERM-NITRO	
AB2	**NOVARTIS**	**0.1 mg/hr**
AB2		**0.2 mg/hr**
AB2		**0.4 mg/hr**
AB2		**0.6 mg/hr**

Figure B

	NITROGLYCERIN	
	Film, Extended Release; Transdermal	
AB2	**HERCON**	**0.2 mg/hr**
AB2		**0.4 mg/hr**
AB2		**0.6 mg/hr**
AB2	**MYLAN**	**0.1 mg/hr**
AB2		**0.2 mg/hr**
AB2		**0.4 mg/hr**
AB2		**0.6 mg/hr**
	Injectable; Injection	
AP	**POHL BOSKAMP**	**5 mg/mL**
AP	**HOECHST MARION**	**5 mg/mL**
AP	**ABBOTT**	**5 mg/mL**

Figure C

52. A prescription calls for Nitro-Dur transdermal patch 0.1 mg/hr. Which of the following transdermal products may be dispensed if substitution is required? (See Figures B & C)
    I. 3M's Minitran 0.1 mg/hr.
    II. Mylan's NTG 0.1 mg/hr.
    III. Novartis's NTG 0.1 mg/hr.
    (A) I only (B) III only (C) I & II only
    (D) II & III only (E) I, II, & III

53. Which of the following companies' 0.2 mg/hr nitroglycerin patches are considered to be interchangeable when substituting? (See Figures B & C)
    I. Hercon Labs
    II. Mylan
    III. Novartis
    (A) I only (B) III only (C) I & II only
    (D) II & III only (E) I, II, & III

54. A prescription order is written "NTG injection 5 mg/mL". Assuming that substitution is permissible, which of the following companies' products could be used? (See Figure C)
    I. Pohl Boskamp
    II. Hoechst Marion
    III. Abbott
    (A) I only (B) III only (C) I & II only
    (D) II & III only (E) I, II, & III

55. A prescription order is written "NTG injection 5mg/mL". Assuming that substitution is NOT permissible, which of the following companies' products could be used? (See Figure C)
    I. Pohl Boskamp
    II. Hoechst Marion
    III. Abbott
    (A) I only (B) III only (C) I & II only
    (D) II & III only (E) I, II, & III

56. A prescription order is written "Tranderm-Nitro 0.4 mg/hr". Assuming that substitution is NOT permissible, which of the following companies' products could be used? (See Figure B)
I. Novartis
II. Mylan
III. Hercon
(A) I only (B) III only (C) I & II only
(D) II & III only (E) I, II, & III

57. A pharmacy carries a complete stock of Nitro-Dur and Minitran patches. In which of the following strengths are these two lines considered bioequivalent? (See Figures B & C)
I. 0.2 mg/hr
II. 0.4 mg/hr
III. 0.8 mg/hr
(A) I only (B) III only (C) I & II only
(D) II & III only (E) I, II, & III

58. Original packages of nitroglycerin that are exempt from the requirements of the Poison Prevention Packaging Act include:
I. oral tablets
II. ointments
III. SL tablets
(A) I only (B) III only (C) I & II only
(D) II & III only (E) I, II, & III

59. Which one of the following dosage forms is least likely to present bioequivalence problems?
(A) capsule (B) IV solution (C) suspension
(D) transdermal patch (E) tablet

60. Certain drug products are exempt from the requirements of therapeutic equivalence because of:
I. their high therapeutic index
II. their use in chemotherapy
III. the grandfather clause

(A) I only (B) III only (C) I & II only
(D) II & III only (E) I, II, & III

61. Which of the following commercial products intended for oral intake need identification codes on the individual units?
I. Nonprescription tablets
II. Prescription tablets
III. Prescription capsules dosage forms
(A) I only (B) III only (C) I & II only
(D) II & III only (E) I, II, & III

62. Which of the following reference sources contain significant information concerning the bioequivalence of drug products?
I. USP/NF
II. USP/DI
III. Orange Book
(A) I only (B) III only (C) I & II only
(D) II & III only (E) I, II, & III

63. Permission to not use a child-resistant closure on a prescription may be made by the
I. pharmacist
II. prescriber
III. patient
(A) I only (B) III only (C) I & II only
(D) II & III only (E) I, II, & III

64. Enforcement of the PPPA is basically under the jurisdiction of the:
(A) Food and Drug Administration (FDA)
(B) Federal Trade Commission (FTC)
(C) Consumer Product Safety Commission (CPSC)
(D) US Justice Department
(E) Health Care Financing Administration (HCFA)

65. In which of the following situations are child-resistant closures NOT required?
    I. When a community pharmacist dispenses fewer than 10 tablets of a drug product
    II. When a hospital pharmacy is filling a prescription for an outpatient
    III. When a hospital pharmacy fills a prescription for an inpatient

    (A) I only (B) III only (C) I & II only
    (D) II & III only (E) I, II, & III

66. Packaging for nonprescription products that is designed to prevent the addition of foreign material into the final product is best described as being:
    (A) tamper-evident (B) tamper-proof
    (C) tamper-resistant (D) hermetically sealed
    (E) air-tight

67. A neighboring community pharmacy requests Alcohol USP/NF from your hospital pharmacy, which has tax-free alcohol. Under what circumstances may you supply the alcohol?
    (A) It is never permissible
    (B) Limiting your sale to not more than one pint
    (C) By making a simple loan of the alcohol
    (D) Any circumstances are permissible
    (E) By charging the pharmacy the purchase price plus the alcohol tax

68. With respect to reimbursement, wheelchairs are classified as being:
    (A) AWP's (B) DME's
    (C) DRG's (D) GRASE
    (E) NDC's

69. The strictest expiration dating for compounded prescriptions is for which of the following dosage forms?
(A) aqueous solutions (B) capsules (C) lotions
(D) nonaqueous solutions (E) ointments

70. The label of a bottle of Ipecac Syrup sold OTC for accidental poisoning must:
I. must have its warnings printed in red ink.
II. contain the telephone number of the regional poison control center.
III. state that the appropriate dose is the entire bottle followed by a full glass of water.
(A) I only (B) III only (C) I & II only
(D) II & III only (E) I, II, & III

71. An orphan drug is one that has
(A) been removed from the market because of toxicity
(B) has been discontinued because of poor sales
(C) provides special economic incentives for the manufacturer
(D) has a low therapeutic index
(E) has been developed and imported from a foreign country

72. Which of the following statements concerning drug recalls is(are) accurate?
I. They occur only after fatalities have occurred.
II. They can be ordered by the FDA.
III. They are voluntary actions by the pharmaceutical manufacturer
(A) I only (B) III only (C) I & II only
(D) II & III only (E) I, II, & III

73. Which of the following effervescent products are usually exempted from the Poison Prevention Packaging Act?
I. aspirin
II. acetaminophen
III. potassium chloride

(A) I only (B) III only (C) I and II only
(D) II and III only (E) I, II, and III

74. The Poison Prevention Packaging Act (PPPA) is intended to protect
    I. young children
    II. geriatric patients
    III. potentially suicidal patients
    (A) I only (B) III only (C) I & II only
    (D) II & III only (E) I, II, & III

75. Which of the following must be imprinted on each commercial oral tablet?
    (A) Company name
    (B) Name and strength of the drug
    (C) A code identifying each of the above
    (D) An expiration date
    (E) Date of manufacturing

76. Federal guidelines indicate that the pharmacist should indicate the date on which a prescription refill is dispensed
    (A) on the front of the prescription
    (B) on the back of the prescription
    (C) on the prescription label
    (D) in a special refill log book
    (E) on the counseling sheet given to the patient

77. Under what circumstance(s) may a pharmacist NOT refuse to accept or fill a prescription:
    (A) The prescription is suspected to be either forged or fictitiously written.
    (B) The patient is known to be HIV positive.
    (C) The pharmacist believes that he will be violating the law by filling the prescription.
    (D) The drug or drug product is not in stock.
    (E) The pharmacist believes that the drug product may be harmful to the patient.

78. Prescription drug package inserts include all of the following types of information EXCEPT:
(A) adverse reactions
(B) contraindications
(C) symptoms and treatment of overdosing
(D) AWP's
(E) date of most recent revision of the labeling

79. Which one of the following types of information found in the prescription drug package insert is most critical in determining whether to dispense a certain drug to a specific patient?
(A) adverse reactions
(B) contraindications
(C) cautions
(D) warnings
(E) indications

80. When refilling a prescription that requires a child-resistant container, the pharmacist must always replace which of the following?
I. The plastic closure
II. The plastic container
III. The glass container
(A) I only (B) III only (C) I & II only
(D) II & III only (E) I, II, & III

81. Which of the following categories of pregnancy warnings is the most severe?
(A) Category A
(B) Category D
(C) Category III
(D) Category X
(E) Category NR

82. Under which one of the following circumstances may a pharmacist refuse to fill a prescription?

(A) The quantity of the controlled drug has been changed.
(B) The pharmacist does not know the patient.
(C) The patient is an alcoholic.
(D) The prescription was written a week ago.
(E) The prescriber is from another city.

83. According to the present DSHEA, an herbal product such as Saw Palmetto may be labeled to state:
(A) cures prostatitis
(B) help treat prostatitis
(C) for the prostate
(D) helps in prevention of prostate cancer
(E) will return the prostate to normal size

84. Every new drug placed on the market will have a designated
I. generic name
II. tradename
III. brandname
(A) I only (B) III only (C) I and II only
(D) II and III only (E) I, II, and III

85. In which of the following locations would you NOT find pharmaceutical manufacturer's drug samples?
I. hospital pharmacy
II. physician's office
III. chain or community pharmacy
(A) I only (B) III only (C) I and II only
(D) II and III only (E) I, II, and III

86. What number is given to the clinical trial phase that consists of post-marketing surveillance of a drug that was recently introduced onto the market?
(A) 1 (B) 2 (C) 3 (D) 4 (E) 5

87. With respect to pregnancy warnings, category D indicates that the drug
    - (A) is safe for 98% of all females during pregnancy.
    - (B) should not be used during the first trimester.
    - (C) should be administered only if the potential benefits are acceptable despite the potential risks.
    - (D) should not be used during the pregnancy.
    - (E) does not pose any danger to either the mother or fetus.

88. Which one of the following laws first required the statement "Caution: Federal law prohibits dispensing without a prescription" on drug product packaging?
    - (A) Durham-Humphrey Amendment
    - (B) FD and C Act of 1938
    - (C) Kefauver-Harris Amendment
    - (D) Prescription Drug Marketing Act
    - (E) Pure Food and Drug Act of 1906

89. Adverse effects involving which of the following should be reported to MedWatch?
    - I. controlled substances
    - II. medical devices
    - III. vaccines

    (A) I only (B) III only (C) I & II only
    (D) II & III only (E) I, II & III

90. Which government body is responsible for funding and overseeing state Medicaid programs?

    (A) DHHS (B) FDA (C) HCFA
    (D) NABP (E) USP/NF

91. A product that contains not more than 1.8 g of codeine per 100 mL is considered to be in Schedule

    (A) I (B) II (C) III (D) IV (E) V

92. The label of a bottle of Ipecac Syrup sold OTC for accidental poisoning must:
    I. state that the appropriate dose is the contents of the entire bottle followed by a full glass of water.
    II. provide the telephone number of a poison control center.
    III. must have its warnings printed in red ink.
    (A) I only (B) III only (C) I & II only
    (D) II & III only (E) I, II, & III

93. Dronabinol is a Schedule II controlled substance that is related most closely to
    (A) cocaine (B) morphine (C) LSD
    (D) marijuana (E) methylphenidate

94. A pharmacy develops and prepares batches of 5,000 sustained-release capsules similar to a commercially available product, but at a lower price. The pharmacy may be cited for this activity based upon:
    I. The capsule formula may be considered a new drug.
    II. The preparation of 5,000 capsules may be considered manufacturing.
    III. The failure to following GMP's.
    (A) I only (B) III only (C) I & II only
    (D) II & III only (E) I, II, & III

95. Hospital inpatients receiving oral estrogen therapy must receive patient package inserts:
    (A) every day
    (B) only with the first dose
    (C) at least every 30 days
    (D) at least every 7 days
    (E) only at the first dose and when being discharged

96. Which one of the following acronyms is most closely associated with health care reimbursement?
(A) DEA (B) DRG (C) GMP
(D) JCAHO (E) PPI

97. Hospitalized patients that are part of a comprehensive narcotic treatment program may receive methadone doses by which of the following routes?
I. Oral
II. Parenteral
III. Transdermal
(A) I only (B) III only (C) I & II only
(D) II & III only (E) I, II, & III

98. Two generic companies manufacture a specific drug in several dosage forms. Which one of the dosage forms is most likely to present problems with bioequivalence?
(A) aerosol
(B) capsule
(C) oral solution
(D) parenteral solution
(E) tablet

99. The National Drug Code (NDC) consists of a series of
(A) letters only
(B) letters and numbers
(C) numbers only
(D) numbers and symbols
(E) symbols only

100. The first series of digits in the NDC for a drug product represents the:
(A) drug name
(B) drug strength
(C) manufacturer
(D) package size
(E) therapeutic use

101. The acronym, DUR, is most closely associated with which of the following?
  (A) drug clinical trials
  (B) Medicare reimbursement
  (C) MedWatch
  (D) drug nomenclature
  (E) patient counseling

102. Schedule III, IV, or V controlled substances may be refilled
  I. not more than 6 times
  II. not more than for a 6 month period
  III. only if authorized by the prescriber
  (A) I only (B) III only (C) I & II only
  (D) II & III only (E) I, II, & III

103. The drug patent of an innovator company has expired. Which one of the following must a second drug company submit to place a generic form of the drug product onto the market?
  (A) abbreviated new drug application
  (B) investigational new drug application
  (C) new drug application
  (D) generic drug application
  (E) supplemental new drug application

104. Hospitals that plan on using large quantities of tax-free grain alcohol should obtain which one of the following forms?
  (A) ATF 11 (B) ATF 222 (C) ATF 1447
  (D) DEA 222 (E) DEA 1447

105. Oral authorization for additional refills on a schedule III prescription are acceptable as long as
  I. the total quantity authorized does not exceed five refills within a six-month period from the date of issue of the original prescription.
  II. the quantity of each additional refill authorized is not greater than the quantity authorized for the initial filling of the prescription.

III. the pharmacist gets a "cover" prescription from the prescriber within 7 days of the oral authorization.

(A) I only (B) III only (C) I & II only
(D) II & III only (E) I, II, & III

106. Which one of the following actions is permissible in a hospital that has tax-free alcohol?
(A) dispensing to inpatients in the form of a tonic
(B) loan pint quantities to community pharmacies
(C) loan pint quantities to other hospitals
(D) sell pint quantities to community pharmacies
(E) sell pint quantities to physician offices

107. The statement "Rx only" does NOT need to appear on the packaging of
(A) orphan drugs
(B) controlled substances
(C) legend drugs
(D) OTC products
(E) injectable products

108. Who is responsible for the retrospective drug utilization reviews established by OBRA 90?
(A) all dispensing pharmacists
(B) consultant pharmacists
(C) each state
(D) hospital pharmacies
(E) individual community pharmacies

109. Which of the following statements is (are) true with respect to the National Drug Code?
I. NDC must be imprinted on tablets.
II. NDC must be imprinted on capsules.
III. All prescription drug products marketed in the US must have NDC's.

(A) I only (B) III only (C) I and II only
(D) II and III only (E) I, II, and III

110. The main responsibility for oversight of prescription drug advertising rests with the
(A) FDA (B) FTC (C) HCFA
(D) DEA (E) USP/NF

111. A drug product consisting of tablets may be declared adulterated for all of the following reasons EXCEPT:
(A) active drug has undergone partial decomposition
(B) contains an unapproved color additive
(C) does not indicate number of tablets present
(D) inactive ingredient has undergone partial decomposition
(E) manufactured in a plant that fails to meet GMP's

112. Based upon the Federal Anti-drug Abuse Act of 1988, a pharmacy employee who is convicted of criminal possession of illegal drugs must:
(A) inform his/her employer within 5 days of the conviction
(B) inform his/her employer within one year of the conviction
(C) volunteer to enter a drug rehabilitation program
(D) volunteer to perform at least 1000 hours of community service
(E) resign his/her position from a pharmacy

113. Excipients included in pharmaceutical dosage forms are usually found on which of the following lists?
(A) DSHEA (B) GRAS (C) HPLC
(D) Top 200 (E) UPS

114. Which one of the following pieces of information is NOT encoded into a drug product's NDC?
(A) drug name
(B) manufacturer
(C) product's expiration date
(D) package size
(E) strength of a tablet

115. The organization responsible for the accreditation of many health institutions such as hospitals is the:
(A) APhA (B) ASHP (C) HHS
(D) FTC (E) JCAHO

116. A drug product consisting of tablets may be declared misbranded under all of the following guidelines EXCEPT:
(A) does not meet assay limits
(B) does not indicate number of tablets present
(C) official names of certain ingredients not used
(D) name and location of manufacturer is missing
(E) portion of the label is misleading

117. Which form must a community pharmacy use to purchase grain alcohol for compounding?
(A) ATF 11 (B) ATF 222 (C) DEA 222
(D) DEA 23a (E) FDA 23a

118. The Marketing Act of 1987 guarantees a company that discovers, patents, and develops a new drug exclusive marketing rights for up to:
(A) 20 years (B) 10 years (C) 17 years
(D) 50 years (E) 100 years

119. When a Schedule II prescription is partially filled for an LTCF patient
I. the prescription is valid not more than 60 days from the issue date.
II. the pharmacist must write "LTCF patient" on the prescription
III. the total quantity dispensed cannot exceed 100 dosage units
(A) I only (B) III only (C) I & II only
(D) II & III only (E) I, II, & III

120. Which of the following are exempt from registration under the Controlled Substance Act?
I. A U.S. Army physician
II. A U.S. Public Health Service physician
III. A foreign-trained physician
(A) I only (B) III only (C) I & II only
(D) II & III only (E) I, II, & III

121. The statement "Caution: Federal law prohibits the transfer of this drug to any person other than the patient for whom it was prescribed" is not required for
I. controlled substances dispensed for use in "blinded" clinical investigations.
II. dispensing Schedule V drugs.
III. dispensing controlled substances to be administered to a patient in an institution.
(A) I only (B) III only (C) I & II only
(D) II & III only (E) I, II, & III

122. The total number of digits in the NDC numbers present on a pharmaceutical package may be:
(A) 2 or 3 (B) 5 or 6 (C) 8 or 9
(D) 10 or 11 (E) 15 to 16

123. Which of the following is true about DEA Form 222?
I. If it contains incorrect information the supplier may correct it and initial the correction.
II. If an order cannot be filled by a supplier the form must be returned to the purchaser.
III. If any forms are lost, the loss must be reported to DEA.
(A) I only (B) III only (C) I & II only
(D) II & III only (E) I, II, & III

124. A hospital that has two 55-gallon drums of tax-free grain alcohol must:
(A) maintain a running inventory of the volume
(B) inventory the stock every month
(C) inventory the stock every 6 months

(D) report the amount remaining to the ATF every six months
(E) take a year-end inventory

125. The term "Grandfathered" refers to drugs that were marketed before passage of the:
(A) FD & C Act of 1938
(B) Durham-Humphrey Act
(C) DSHEA
(D) Kefauver-Harris Amendment of 1962
(E) Poison Prevention Act

126. A statement that a specific OTC product has a tamper-evident feature may be placed in any of the following locations EXCEPT on the:
(A) closure
(B) front of the package
(C) back of the package
(D) on the tamper-evident device
(E) under the product name

127. Which of the following drug products must be purchased using a DEA Form 222?
I. Levoprome
II. Demerol
III. Duragesic-50
(A) I only (B) III only (C) I & II only
(D) II & III only (E) I, II, & III

128. Which of the following agents is an anabolic steroid?
I. nandrolone
II. fluticasone
III. hydrocortisone
(A) I only (B) III only (C) I & II only
(D) II & III only (E) I, II, & III

129. "Grandfathered" drugs are
(A) found in the Orange Book as Code A only.
(B) found in the Orange Book as Code B only.
(C) found in the Orange Book as Code AB only.

(D) to be prescribed only by generic name.
(E) often not listed in the Orange Book.

130. A pharmacy that compounds many prescriptions may be cited by the FDA if the volume of its prescriptions being sent to out-of-state is in excess of ____ %.
(A) 2 (B) 5 (C) 10 (D) 20 (E) 50

131. Into how many segments is the NDC number on a pharmaceutical package divided?
(A) 2 (B) 3 (C) 4
(D) 5 (E) greater than 5

132. The first phase of a clinical trial, which evaluates the efficacy of the drug in treating a specific disease, is:
(A) phase I (B) phase II (C) phase III
(D) phase IV (E) phase V

133. The maximum volume of Ipecac Syrup that may be sold without a prescription is:
(A) 15 mL (B) 30 mL (C) 60 mL
(D) 120mL (E) > 120 mL

134. Short-term detoxification treatment is defined as treatment that does not exceed
(A) 24 hours (B) 7 days (C) 30 days
(D) 90 days (E) 180 days

135. Which of the following clinical trial stages is conducted exclusively in healthy humans?
(A) phase I (B) phase II (C) phase III
(D) phase IV (E) phase I and II

136. Which of the following drugs are considered to be "Basic Class" drugs under the Controlled Substances Act?
I. dextroamphetamine
II. codeine
III. phenobarbital
(A) I only (B) III only (C) I & II only
(D) II & III only (E) I, II, & III

137. A customer enters your pharmacy and requests 25 x 260 mg quinine tablets. Which of the following responses by the pharmacist would be appropriate?
I. Quinine tablets can no longer be sold over-the-counter.
II. OTC quinine is considered to be unsafe for the prevention of malaria.
III. OTC quinine is considered ineffective for the treatment of nocturnal leg cramps.
(A) I only (B) III only (C) I and II only
(D) II and III only (E) I, II, and III

138. Which of the following are mid-level practitioners?
I. Nurse Practitioners
II. Nurse Midwives
III. Podiatrists
(A) I only (B) III only (C) I & II only
(D) II & III only (E) I, II, & III

139. Under which of the following circumstances may Ipecac Syrup be sold without a prescription?
I. for future potential use during accidental poisoning
II. only if the household does not have small children
III. if the purchaser signs a pharmacy log book for the sale
(A) I only (B) III only (C) I & II only
(D) II & III only (E) I, II, & III

140. Which of the following DEA forms are used to apply for registration?
I. Form 222
II. Form 222a
III. Form 224
(A) I only (B) III only (C) I & II only
(D) II & III only (E) I, II, & III

141. Which of the following are Schedule II controlled substances?
   I. sufentanyl
   II. psilocyn
   III. chloral hydrate
   (A) I only (B) III only (C) I & II only
   (D) II & III only (E) I, II, & III

142. Phenobarbital is a drug that is classified as a(n)
   (A) Schedule III drug (B) Schedule IV drug
   (C) Schedule V drug (D) non-controlled drug
   (E) OTC drug

143. All of the following drugs fall into the category of "Grandfathered Drugs" EXCEPT:
   (A) ampicillin
   (B) ephedrine
   (C) epinephrine
   (D) phenobarbital
   (E) thyroid

144. Which of the following are Schedule I controlled substances?
   I. mescaline
   II. peyote
   III. heroin
   (A) I only (B) III only (C) I & II only
   (D) II & III only (E) I, II, & III

145. Which of the products listed below would be considered to be Schedule III controlled substances?
   I. A product that contains 90 mg of codeine per dose
   II. A product that contains 15 mg of hydrocodone per dose
   III. A product that contains 2.5 mg of diphenoxylate and 25 mcg of atropine sulfate per dose
   (A) I only (B) III only (C) I & II only
   (D) II & III only (E) I, II, & III

146. Primary responsibility for oversight of nonprescription drug advertising rests with the
(A) FDA (B) FTC (C) HCFA
(D) DEA (E) USP/NF

147. Partial filling of a schedule IV controlled substance prescription is permissible, provided that
I. each partial filling is recorded.
II. the total quantity dispensed in all partial fillings does not exceed the total quantity prescribed.
III. the total price charged for the partial fillings does not exceed the total price the patient would have paid with a complete filling of the prescription.
(A) I only (B) III only (C) I & II only
(D) II & III only (E) I, II, & III

148. When a pharmacist conducts a controlled substance inventory, which of the following must be included?
I. Drugs stored in a warehouse for the registrant at a different location
II. Drugs ordered by a customer but not yet paid for.
III. All controlled substances dispensed over the past 30 days.
(A) I only (B) III only (C) I & II only
(D) II & III only (E) I, II, & III

149. Which of the following are Schedule IV controlled substances?
I. mazindol
II. fenfluramine
III. buprenorphine
(A) I only (B) III only (C) I & II only
(D) II & III only (E) I, II, & III

150. A "Listed Chemical" is defined by the Controlled Substances Act as any chemical that is
(A) a controlled substance
(B) listed in the USP/NF

(C) listed in the USP DI
(D) used in manufacturing a controlled substance
(E) listed in the Orange Book

151. Percogesic is an example of a product that is
(A) in Schedule II (B) in Schedule III
(C) in Schedule IV (D) in Schedule V
(E) not a controlled substance

152. Which of the following are Schedule II controlled substances?
I. morphine
II. fentanyl
III. secobarbital
(A) I only (B) III only (C) I & II only
(D) II & III only (E) I, II, & III

153. The original portion of the Form 222 is eventually kept on file by the
(A) DEA (B) purchaser (C) FDA
(D) supplier (E) prescriber

154. Copy 3 of DEA Form 222 is eventually kept by the
(A) DEA (B) supplier (C) purchaser
(D) prescriber (E) FDA

155. Which of the following barbiturates are classified as Schedule II controlled substances?
I. amobarbital
II. pentobarbital
III. butabarbital
(A) I only (B) III only (C) I & II only
(D) II & III only (E) I, II, & III

156. Which of the following is true about DEA Form 222?
I. It may be used by any pharmacy in the same chain
II. It may be partially filled by the supplier
III. A physician may use it to order Schedule II controlled substances

(A) I only (B) III only (C) I & II only
(D) II & III only (E) I, II, & III

157. Which of the following products are Schedule III controlled substances?
   I. Demerol tablets
   II. Empirin with Codeine #3
   III. Tylenol with Codeine #1
   (A) I only (B) III only (C) I & II only
   (D) II & III only (E) I, II, & III

158. DEA form 222a is used
   (A) to order Schedule II controlled substances
   (B) to order all controlled substances
   (C) to requisition Form 222
   (D) to return unused controlled substances
   (E) to register a practitioner with DEA

159. A filled DEA Form 222 must be kept
   I. by the supplier for 2 years
   II. by the purchaser for 3 years
   III. by the DEA for 10 years
   (A) I only (B) III only (C) I & II only
   (D) II & III only (E) I, II, & III

160. Which of the following is true of DEA Form 222?
   I. It is used to order Schedule II controlled substances
   II. Only one product may be ordered on each line of the form
   III. May be used to order syringes and hypodermic needles.
   (A) I only (B) III only (C) I & II only
   (D) II & III only (E) I, II, & III

161. Controlled substances prescriptions may be issued by prescribers
    I. to obtain controlled substances for dispensing in their office
    II. to prescribe drugs to be used by a patient for narcotic detoxification
    III to prescribe controlled substances for a patient with chronic pain.
    (A) I only (B) III only (C) I & II only
    (D) II & III only (E) I, II, & III

162. Controlled substance prescriptions
    I. may be written by typewriter (except for the prescriber's signature).
    II. must have the name of the physician printed, stamped, typed, or hand-printed on it.
    III. may be prepared by an agent of the prescriber for the prescriber's signature
    (A) I only (B) III only (C) I & II only
    (D) II & III only (E) I, II, & III

163. Which of the following are Schedule IV controlled substances?
    I. flurazepam
    II. halazepam
    III. zolpidem
    (A) I only (B) III only (C) I & II only
    (D) II & III only (E) I, II, & III

164. Any physician is permitted to
    I. prescribe drugs to relieve acute narcotic withdrawal symptoms
    II. administer drugs to relieve acute narcotic withdrawal symptoms
    III. administer drugs to provide narcotic drug-dependent patients with maintenance treatment
    (A) I only (B) III only (C) I & II only
    (D) II & III only (E) I, II, & III

165. Which of the following is true of DEA Form 222?
    I. May be used to transfer Schedule II drugs from one pharmacy to another.
    II. May be used to return Schedule II drugs to the supplier.
    III. It must contain the name and address of the supplier from whom schedule II controlled substances are being ordered.

    (A) I only (B) III only (C) I & II only
    (D) II & III only (E) I, II, & III

166. Oral orders for Schedule II drugs may be accepted and dispensed by a pharmacist
    I. in an emergency situation.
    II. only if the physician is more than 100 miles away from the pharmacy.
    III. if a patient is a regular customer of the pharmacy.

    (A) I only (B) III only (C) I & II only
    (D) II & III only (E) I, II, & III

167. Schedule II prescriptions
    I. may only be refilled once
    II. may be partially filled under certain conditions
    III. written for a hospice patient may be faxed to a pharmacy

    (A) I only (B) III only (C) I & II only
    (D) II & III only (E) I, II, & III

168. A pharmacist may partially fill a Schedule II prescription
    I. and the remaining portion of the prescription may be filled within 72 hr of the first partial fill.
    II. if the pharmacist does not have enough medication in stock to completely fill the prescription.
    III. if the patient only wants some of the medication prescribed

    (A) I only (B) III only (C) I & II only
    (D) II & III only (E) I, II, & III

169. A faxed Schedule II prescription from the prescriber to a pharmacy is permitted
   I. at any time as long as it is followed by a written "cover" prescription.
   II. if the patient is a resident of a Long Term Care Facility
   III. if the patient is a hospice patient.
   (A) I only (B) III only (C) I & II only
   (D) II & III only (E) I, II, & III

170. To be admitted to a comprehensive maintenance program, a narcotic-dependent individual must have been physiologically dependent on narcotics for at least
   (A) 30 days (B) 90 days (C) 180 days
   (D) 12 months (E) 18 months

171. Which of the following is/are NOT required to be on a prescription for a controlled substance?
   I. DEA number of the practitioner
   II. The date on which the prescription was signed
   III. The date of birth of the patient
   (A) I only (B) III only (C) I & II only
   (D) II & III only (E) I, II, & III

172. Which of the following is true?
   I. Original schedule III, IV, or V prescriptions may be transferred from one pharmacy to another for the purpose of refill dispensing.
   II. Information from schedule III, IV, or V prescriptions may not be transferred to another pharmacy unless authorized by the prescriber to do so.
   III. Pharmacies electronically sharing a real-time, online database may transfer refills to one another as long as the number of refills transferred does not exceed those authorized by the prescriber or the law.
   (A) I only (B) III only (C) I & II only
   (D) II & III only (E) I, II, & III

173. Which of the following drug products must be purchased by pharmacies using DEA Form 222?
  I. Ritalin
  II. MS Contin
  III. Dalgan
  (A) I only (B) III only (C) I & II only
  (D) II & III only (E) I, II, & III

174. Which of the following is NOT required on the prescription label when the pharmacist fills a controlled substance prescription?
  I. Date of initial filling
  II. Federal "Caution" warning
  III. Number of dosage units dispensed
  (A) I only (B) III only (C) I & II only
  (D) II & III only (E) I, II, & III

175. Which of the following is true of dispensing controlled substance-containing products without a prescription?
  I. Not more than 120mL or 24 dosage units of Robitussin A-C cough medicine may be dispensed in any given 48-hour period.
  II. Not more than 240mL or 48 dosage units of Camphorated Opium Tincture (Paregoric) may be dispensed in any given 48-hour period.
  III. The purchaser must be at least 21 years of age
  (A) I only (B) III only (C) I & II only
  (D) II & III only (E) I, II, & III

176. Schedule III, IV, and V controlled substance prescriptions may be issued to a community pharmacy pursuant to
  I. a fax of a written, signed prescription transmitted by the prescriber to the pharmacy
  II. an oral prescription called in by a prescriber
  III. a written prescription signed by the prescriber
  (A) I only (B) III only (C) I & II only
  (D) II & III only (E) I, II, & III

177. Which of the following is true of Schedule II controlled substances?

  I. They may be dispensed by a community pharmacist only pursuant to a written prescription signed by the practitioner.
  II. They may be administered or dispensed by a physician without a prescription to a patient with chronic pain.
  III. They may be administered by an institutional pharmacist pursuant to an order for immediate administration to the ultimate user.

(A) I only (B) III only (C) I & II only
(D) II & III only (E) I, II, & III

178. Which of the following is true of controlled substance inventories?

  I. Inventories for schedule II controlled substances must be kept separately from all other records of the pharmacy.
  II. Controlled substance inventories must be performed annually.
  III. The registrant must keep inventory records for at least 5 years from the date performed.

(A) I only (B) III only (C) I & II only
(D) II & III only (E) I, II, & III

179. Short-term narcotic detoxification is defined as treatment that is for a period of less than

(A) 30 days (B) 60 days (C) 90 days
(D) 180 days (E) 1 year

180. When conducting a controlled substance inventory, the registrant
    I. must make an exact count of open containers of Schedule II substances.
    II. may estimate the count of a Schedule IV substance in an opened container that originally held 500 tablets.
    III. must make an exact count of all controlled substances in sealed, unopened containers.

    (A) I only (B) III only (C) I & II only
    (D) II & III only (E) I, II, & III

181. When a physician faxes a Schedule II prescription to a pharmacy for a LTCF patient
    I. the pharmacist must call the LTCF to verify the identity of the patient.
    II. the physician must first call the pharmacy to advise them that a fax is being issued.
    III. the original written, signed prescription must be presented to the pharmacist for review prior to the actual dispensing of the controlled fax.

    (A) I only (B) III only (C) I & II only
    (D) II & III only (E) I, II, & III

182. Controlled substance inventories
    I. may be done at any time during the workday.
    II. must be taken at least once each year.
    III. must be made for each registered location.

    (A) I only (B) III only (C) I & II only
    (D) II & III only (E) I, II, & III

183. A hospital pharmacy director is informed that an employee has been convicted of selling cocaine on the street. Which of the following actions may the director take based upon the Federal Anti-drug Abuse Act of 1988?
   - I. warn the employee not to possess or sell illegal drugs in the future
   - II. place a letter of reprimand in the employee's personnel file
   - III. terminate the employment of the individual

   (A) I only (B) III only (C) I and II only
   (D) II and III only (E) I, II, and III

184. Narcotic drugs may be dispensed to treat narcotic dependence in which of the following facilities?
   - I. Any institutional pharmacy
   - II. Any facility with a DEA certified narcotic treatment counselor
   - III. FDA and state approved narcotic treatment programs

   (A) I only (B) III only (C) I & II only
   (D) II & III only (E) I, II, & III

185. Blood and/or urine tests are frequently performed on participants in comprehensive narcotic maintenance treatment programs in order to detect
   - I. drug toxicity
   - II. hepatotoxicity
   - III. continued abuse of drugs

   (A) I only (B) III only (C) I & II only
   (D) II & III only (E) I, II, & III

186. Which of the following is true?
   I. Prescribers must keep records of all controlled substances that they dispense directly to the patient.
   II. Prescribers must keep records of all controlled substances administered in the course of narcotic detoxification treatment.
   III. Prescribers must keep records of all controlled substances that they receive as samples
   (A) I only (B) III only (C) I & II only
   (D) II & III only (E) I, II, & III

187. When a patient begins a comprehensive narcotic treatment program, the first day's dose of methadone must generally not exceed
   (A) 0.5 mg (B) 1 mg (C) 5 mg
   (D) 20 mg (E) 40 mg

188. Which of the following is/are used in the treatment of narcotic dependence?
   I. LAAM
   II. methadone
   III. prostigmine
   (A) I only (B) III only (C) I & II only
   (D) II & III only (E) I, II, & III

189. Chloral hydrate is an example of a drug product in controlled substance schedule
   (A) I (B) II (C) III (D) IV (E) V

190. Which of the following products are NOT controlled substances?
   I. Mepergan
   II. Melphalan
   III. Megestrol acetate
   (A) I only (B) III only (C) I & II only
   (D) II & III only (E) I, II, & III

191. Prescriptions for which of the following controlled substances may be partially filled upon request of the patient:

I. Dilaudid
II. Ritalin
III. Empirin w/codeine #4

(A) I only (B) III only (C) I & II only
(D) II & III only (E) I, II, & III

192. Which of the following are NOT controlled substances?

I. ergotamine tartrate
II. papaverine
III. levorphanol

(A) I only (B) III only (C) I & II only
(D) II & III only (E) I, II, & III

193. Which of the following employees may administer or dispense drugs to patients as part of a narcotic treatment program?

I. Pharmacists
II. Registered nurses
III. Licensed practical nurses

(A) I only (B) III only (C) I & II only
(D) II & III only (E) I, II, & III

194. Pharmacists are required to periodically inventory supplies of which of the following drug products?

I. phenobarbital elixir
II. Entex Liquid
III. Sudafed Plus Liquid

(A) I only (B) III only (C) I & II only
(D) II & III only (E) I, II, & III

195. Which of the following narcotic-dependent patient groups should NOT generally be given LAAM for their treatment?
I. Pregnant women
II. Persons under 18 years of age
III. Individuals who are heroin dependent
(A) I only (B) III only (C) I & II only
(D) II & III only (E) I, II, & III

196. Which of the following drug products must be purchased using a DEA Form 222?
I. Percodan
II. Dilaudid
III. Methadone
(A) I only (B) III only (C) I & II only
(D) II & III only (E) I, II, & III

197. Which of the following drug products are controlled substances?
I. pemoline (Cylert)
II midazolam (Versed)
III. pimozide (Orap)
(A) I only (B) III only (C) I & II only
(D) II & III only (E) I, II, & III

198. Patients treated in an ambulatory care comprehensive narcotic treatment program may receive methadone doses by which of the following routes?
I. oral
II. IM
III. IV
(A) I only (B) III only (C) I & II only
(D) II & III only (E) I, II, & III

199. When LAAM is used to treat narcotic-dependent patients, it should NOT be administered more frequently than
(A) twice daily (B) once daily (C) every other day
(D) twice weekly (E) monthly

200. Which of the following drug products must be ordered using DEA Form 222?
I. methadone
II. sufentanil
III. Percocet
(A) I only (B) III only (C) I & II only
(D) II & III only (E) I, II, & III

201. Methamphetamine is an example of a drug in controlled substance category
(A) I (B) II (C) III (D) IV (E) V

202. The primary objective or charge for individual state boards of pharmacy is the
(A) protection of individual pharmacists
(B) protection of the profession
(C) protection of the general public
(D) enforcement of federal laws
(E) the serving as an intermediary between independent, chain, and institutional pharmacies

203. HCFA is under the jurisdiction of the
(A) Attorney General (B) FDA (C) HHS
(D) JCAHO (E) Dept. of Justice

204. A prescription for methadone is issued for the purpose of managing a patient's narcotic addiction by a physician employed by a narcotic treatment facility. The prescription
I. may be filled in most community pharmacies
II. may be filled only in outpatient institutional pharmacies
III. may not be filled
(A) I only (B) III only (C) I & II only
(D) II & III only (E) I, II, & III

205. Which of the following was the first to require that pharmaceutical manufacturers prove the efficacy of prescription drugs before marketing?
(A) Durham-Humphrey Amendment (1951)
(B) F D & C Act of 1938
(C) Kefauver-Harris Amendment of 1962
(D) Prescription Drug Marketing Act of 1987
(E) Pure Food and Drug Act of 1906

206. Therapeutic substitution is allowed only if an institution is:
(A) nonprofit (B) for profit (C) licensed to do so
(D) using a formulary system
(E) under the supervision of a PharmD

207. A drug that is marketed for the treatment of a relatively rare disease is referred to as a(n):
(A) me-too drug
(B) orphan drug
(C) prodrug
(D) USAN drug
(E) first pass effect drug

208. The USP/NF is best described as a publication that is published by:
(A) the HHS
(B) the FDA
(C) the Pharmaceutical Manufacturer's Association
(D) a coalition of US pharmaceutical companies
(E) an independent organization

209. A pharmacist dispenses a refill for a prescription that originally was written for Adalat but labels the refill as Procardia. This action may be considered:
(A) adulteration
(B) misbranding
(C) misbranding since the generic name was not included
(D) proper since the correct drug was dispensed
(E) negligent only if the prescriber is not informed

210. Evidence indicates that a marketed generic drug product may have a new use for another condition. In order to claim this new indication, a drug manufacturer must:
(A) submit an abbreviated NDA
(B) submit a supplemental NDA
(C) submit a NDA
(D) apply for patent protection
(E) inform the FDA in writing of the revised labeling

211. Filing a supplemental NDA would be appropriate if a pharmaceutical manufacturer wishes to change the
I. excipients included in a capsule formulation
II. shape of a tablet
III. existing tablet from a TID to a once-a-day extended release tablet
(A) I only (B) III only (C) I & II only
(D) II & III only (E) I, II, & III

212. The advertising to the general public of OTC drugs is basically under the regulatory responsibilities of the:
(A) FDA only (B) FDA and FTC (C) FTC only
(D) DEA (E) HCFA

213. A cosmetic company begins marketing of a facial cream that claims to reverse facial wrinkles. This claim may be legally challenged by the:
(A) FDA only (B) FDA and FTC (C) FTC only
(D) DEA (E) HCFA

214. According to Federal law, a pharmacist must include which of the following on a prescription label?
I. name of the dispensing pharmacy
II. address of the dispensing pharmacy
III. name of the dispensing pharmacist
(A) I only (B) III only (C) I & II only
(D) II & III only (E) I, II, & III

215. According to Federal law, a pharmacist must include which of the following on a prescription label?
   I. expiration date from the manufacturer's label
   II. the name of the manufacturer
   III. a prescription serial number
   (A) I only (B) III only (C) I & II only
   (D) II & III only (E) I, II, & III

216. A physician shares with your pharmacy a topical moisturizing formula which contains a prescription drug. Which of the following would be appropriate actions for your pharmacy to take?
   I. Fill prescriptions written by the physician for 120 g of this formula.
   II. Prepare a pound of the formula in anticipation of additional prescriptions or refills.
   III. Prepare 50 x 120 g of the formula for sale from the physician's office.
   (A) I only (B) III only (C) I & II only
   (D) II & III only (E) I, II, & III

217. Which of the following actions is (are) not allowed in a community pharmacy with respect to prescription drug samples?
   I. storing
   II. ordering based upon a specific prescriber's request
   III. dispensing upon receipt of a prescription
   (A) I only (B) III only (C) I & II only
   (D) II & III only (E) I, II, & III

218. The purchasing agent of your hospital suggests that the hospital purchase a two-year's supply of a popular antibiotic at a special price. Which of the following are legal activities?
   I. purchase of that quantity of the antibiotic
   II. sell a portion of the antibiotic to another area hospital
   III. sell a portion of the antibiotic to a community pharmacy

(A) I only (B) III only (C) I & II only
(D) II & III only (E) I, II, & III

219. Uses for tax-free alcohol purchased by a hospital may include:
I. incorporation into formulas for inpatient orders
II. incorporation into prescriptions for recently discharged patients
III. selling of small amounts to independent pharmacies based upon their immediate prescription needs
(A) I only (B) III only (C) I & II only
(D) II & III only (E) I, II, & III

220. The classification of drugs into controlled substance schedules by the federal government is based upon the drug's
I. toxicity
II. therapeutic index
III. potential for abuse and dependence
(A) I only (B) III only (C) I & II only
(D) II & III only (E) I, II, & III

221. The authority for determining the schedule for a potentially new controlled substance belongs to the:
(A) Director of the FDA
(B) President of the US
(C) Director of the DEA
(D) Attorney General of the US
(E) Director of HHS

222. Who must be registered with the DEA in order for a hospital pharmacy to dispense controlled substances?
I. the hospital pharmacy
II. the chief pharmacist
III. every pharmacist who dispenses on a regular basis
(A) I only (B) III only (C) I & II only
(D) II & III only (E) I, II, & III

223. The minimum requirements that a community pharmacist must follow when filling a controlled substance prescriptions written for an outpatient by a hospital resident is that
I. the hospital must have a DEA number
II. the resident must have a DEA number
III. the drug belongs to either Schedule III or IV
(A) I only (B) III only (C) I & II only
(D) II & III only (E) I, II, & III

224. Based upon federal law, which of the following schedules of controlled substances may be dispersed throughout the prescription drug stock of a community pharmacy?
I. Schedule II's
II. Schedule III's
III. Schedule IV and V's
(A) I only (B) III only (C) I & II only
(D) II & III only (E) I, II, & III

225. When inspecting a chain pharmacy, a DEA inspector may audit which of the following records?
I. prescription files
II. invoices for controlled substances
III. financial records of prescription sales and profits
(A) I only (B) III only (C) I & II only
(D) II & III only (E) I, II, & III

226. Which of the following may a nurse in a doctor's office perform, with the prescriber's permission, with regard to a Schedule III prescription?
I. write the prescription and sign the prescriber's name
II. write the prescription except for the drug name, strength, quantity and prescriber's name
III. write the entire prescription except for signing the prescriber's name
(A) I only (B) III only (C) I & II only
(D) II & III only (E) I, II, & III

227. After dispensing prescriptions for several months for a Schedule II analgesic, the pharmacist realizes that the patient with severe pain from bone cancer is addicted to the drug. Which one of the following actions is the most appropriate for the pharmacist?
(A) report the situation to the state board of pharmacy
(B) report the situation to the state medical board
(C) report the situation to the DEA
(D) refuse to fill any further prescriptions
(E) continue to fill the prescriptions

228. Which one of the following designations for drug products that require a prescription in the United States has replaced the designation "Caution: Federal law prohibits dispensing without a prescription"?
(A) "Do not dispense without a prescription."
(B) "Do not transfer to a third party."
(C) "Federal law prohibits use by anyone other than the original patient."
(D) "Rx only"
(E) "Legend drug"

229. Which of the following categories of drugs require the above legend?
I. noncontrolled prescription drugs
II. Schedule II controlled drugs
III. Schedule III and IV controlled drugs
(A) I only (B) III only (C) I & II only
(D) II & III only (E) I, II, & III

230. The statement, "Caution: Federal law prohibits the transfer of this drug to any person other than the person for whom it was prescribed" is required on prescription containers for which of the following categories of drugs?
I. Schedule II
II. Schedule III
III. Schedule IV
(A) I only (B) III only (C) I & II only
(D) II & III only (E) I, II, & III

231. Which of the following are permissible when taking a controlled substance inventory?
 I. assistance of a technician to count tablets
 II. use of a tape recorder
 III. permanent storage of the inventory on a tape recorder
 (A) I only (B) III only (C) I & II only
 (D) II & III only (E) I, II, & III

232. Which of the following items must be ordered from a wholesaler on DEA order form 222?
 I. morphine HCl injection 10 mL vials (10 mg/mL)
 II. meperidine HCl tablets 50 mg
 III. diazepam tablets 10 mg
 (A) I only (B) III only (C) I & II only
 (D) II & III only (E) I, II, & III

233. The requirement that pharmacists must offer to counsel patients concerning their prescriptions was included in which of the following congressional actions?
 (A) Durham-Humphrey Amendment of 1951
 (B) F,D & C Act of 1938
 (C) Kefauver-Harris Amendment of 1962
 (D) Prescription Drug Marketing Act of 1987
 (E) Omnibus Reconcilation Act of 1990

234. Which of the following actions should a pharmacist take if a patient refuses to be counseled about a new prescription?
 I. dispense the prescription but inform the prescriber that counseling was refused
 II. refuse to dispense the prescription
 III. dispense the prescription but note in the prescription files that counseling was refused
 (A) I only (B) III only (C) I & II only
 (D) II & III only (E) I, II, & III

235. Which portion of the Federal counseling regulations must be performed by a committee appointed within each individual state?
I. retrospective review
II. prospective review
III. meta-analysis review
(A) I only (B) III only (C) I & II only
(D) II & III only (E) I, II, & III

236. Which of the following is NOT required on the label of unit dose packages prepared in a hospital?
(A) name of the drug
(B) beyond-use expiration dating
(C) manufacturer's expiration date
(D) strength of drug
(E) control number

237. Which one of the following types of information is useful but not mandatory on the labels of OTC products?
(A) name of manufacturer
(B) address of manufacturer
(C) net contents
(D) NDC number
(E) adequate directions for use

238. The recent discontinuation of use of phenylpropranolamine in OTC products is best described as a:
(A) Class I recall
(B) Class II recall
(C) Class III recall
(D) misbranded product
(E) voluntary discontinuation

239. Which organization is primarily responsible for evaluating the safety and effectiveness of drugs used in veterinary practices?
(A) FDA (B) FTC (C) SPCA
(D) humane society (E) HCFA

240. A pharmacist confides in his hospital's chief pharmacist that he has tested positive for HIV. Which of the following statements is(are) true?

I. The pharmacist may be terminated due to a potentially contagious condition

II. The pharmacist's access to the preparation of parenteral admixtures may be limited.

III. The pharmacist may be considered disabled under the Americans with Disabilities Act.

(A) I only (B) III only (C) I & II only
(D) II & III only (E) I, II, & III

241. Which of the following statements on a cranberry extract label would be acceptable under DSHEA regulations?

I. To reduce E coli counts during a UTI

II. To reduce the incidence and duration of UTI's

III. To help maintain a healthy urinary tract in females

(A) I only (B) III only (C) I & II only
(D) II & III only (E) I, II, & III

242. Which of the following reference sources depict selected laws and regulations especially for controlled substances?

(A) Facts and Comparisons
(B) Physician's Desk Reference
(C) USP DI Volume I
(D) USP DI Volume II
(E) USP DI Volume III

243. Which of the following OTC products must be in a tamper-resistant package?

I. contact lens solution

II. hair shampoo

III. topical lotion

(A) I only (B) III only (C) I & II only
(D) II & III only (E) I, II, & III

244. Running inventories are required of pharmacies for which of the following?

I. Schedule II through IV controlled substances
II. Schedule II controlled substances
III. Tax-free Alcohol

(A) I only (B) III only (C) I & II only
(D) II & III only (E) I, II & III

245. Which of the following would NOT violate the Sherman Antitrust Act?

I. A chain pharmacy purchases the last independent pharmacy in a small city.
II. The independent pharmacy owners vote at their monthly meeting to establish a minimum prescription price of $4.00.
III. A group of independent pharmacies decide to boycott Medicaid prescriptions.

(A) I only (B) III only (C) I & II only
(D) II & III only (E) I, II & III

246. Which of the following testosterone products are classified as Schedule III controlled substances?

I. Testoderm
II. Depo-Testosterone
III. Testoderm TTS

(A) I only (B) III only (C) I & II only
(D) II & III only (E) I, II & III

247. Which of the following drugs are classified as Schedule III controlled substances?

I. ketamine II. thalidomide III. oxytocin

(A) I only (B) III only (C) I & II only
(D) II & III only (E) I, II & III

248. Refills are not allowed for which one of the following drugs?
(A) ProSom (B) MS Contin (C) Versed
(D) Ultram (E) Zydone

249. Drug products that are classified as C IV's include:
I. estazolam (ProSom)
II. midazolam (Versed)
III. tramadol (Ultram)
(A) I only (B) III only (C) I & II only
(D) II & III only (E) I, II & III

250. To which schedule of controlled substances does zaleplon (Sonata) belong?
(A) II
(B) III
(C) IV
(D) V
(E) Rx only but not a controlled substance

Answers to Sample Questions

1.	C	34.	C	67.	A	100.	C
2.	E	35.	E	68.	B	101.	E
3.	E	36.	E	69.	A	102.	D
4.	B	37.	D	70.	A	103.	A
5.	B	38.	C	71.	C	104.	C
6.	C	39.	C	72.	B	105.	C
7.	B	40.	A	73.	E	106.	A
8.	D	41.	C	74.	A	107.	D
9.	B	42.	D	75.	C	108.	C
10.	B	43.	B	76.	B	109.	B
11.	A	44.	A	77.	B	110.	A
12.	B	45.	B	78.	D	111.	C
13.	A	46.	D	79.	B	112.	A
14.	C	47.	E	80.	C	113.	B
15.	B	48.	C	81.	D	114.	C
16.	E	49.	B	82.	A	115.	E
17.	D	50.	E	83.	C	116.	A
18.	B	51.	B	84.	A	117.	A
19.	C	52.	A	85.	B	118.	A
20.	B	53.	E	86.	D	119.	C
21.	D	54.	E	87.	C	120.	C
22.	D	55.	E	88.	A	121.	E
23.	E	56.	A	89.	C	122.	D
24.	C	57.	C	90.	C	123.	D
25.	D	58.	D	91.	C	124.	A
26.	C	59.	B	92.	B	125.	A
27.	C	60.	B	93.	D	126.	D
28.	C	61.	E	94.	E	127.	D
29.	C	62.	D	95.	C	128.	A
30.	E	63.	D	96.	B	129.	E
31.	A	64.	C	97.	C	130.	B
32.	A	65.	B	98.	A	131.	B
33.	D	66.	A	99.	C	132.	B

133. B
134. C
135. A
136. C
137. E
138. C
139. A
140. B
141. A
142. B
143. A
144. E
145. C
146. B
147. C
148. C
149. C
150. D
151. E
152. E
153. D
154. C
155. C
156. D
157. D
158. C
159. A
160. C
161. B
162. E
163. E
164. C
165. E
166. A
167. D
168. C
169. D
170. D
171. B
172. B
173. C
174. B
175. C
176. E
177. E
178. A
179. A
180. E
181. B
182. B
183. E
184. B
185. B
186. C
187. E
188. C
189. D
190. D
191. B
192. C
193. E
194. A
195. C
196. E
197. C
198. A
199. C
200. E
201. B
202. C
203. C
204. B
205. C
206. D
207. B
208. E
209. B
210. A
211. C
212. C
213. B
214. C
215. B
216. C
217. E
218. A
219. A
220. B
221. D
222. A
223. A
224. E
225. C
226. B
227. E
228. D
229. E
230. E
231. C
232. C
233. E
234. B
235. A
236. C
237. D
238. E
239. A
240. B
241. B
242. E
243. A
244. B
245. D
246. E
247. A
248. B
249. C
250. C

Section N

U.S. Boards of Pharmacy

Alabama State Board of Pharmacy
Jerry Moore, Exec. Dir.
1 Perimeter Park South
Suite 425
Birmingham, AL 35243
205/967-0130

Alaska Board of Pharmacy
Debora Stovern
Licensing Examiner
P.O. Box 110806,
Juneau, AK 99811-0806
907/465-2589

Arizona State Board of Pharmacy
Llyn A. Lloyd
Executive Director
4425 W. Olive Avenue, Suite 140
Glendale, AZ 85302
623/463-2727

Arkansas State Board of Pharmacy
Charles S. Campbell
Executive Director
101 E. Capitol, Suite 218,
Little Rock, AR 72201
501/682-0190

California State Board of Pharmacy
Patricia F. Harris
Executive Officer400 R Street, Suite 4070
Sacramento, CA 95814
916/445-5014

Colorado State Board of Pharmacy
Susan L. Warren
Program Administrator
1560 Broadway, Suite 1310
Denver, CO 80202
303/894-7750

Connecticut Commission of Pharmacy
Michelle Sylvestre, Board Administrator
State Office Building, 165 Capitol Avenue, Room 147
Hartford, CT 06106
860/713-6070

Delaware State Board of Pharmacy
David W. Dryden
Executive Secretary
P.O. Box 637
Dover, DE 19901
302/739-4798

District of Columbia Board of Pharmacy
Barbara Hagans
Contact Representative
825 N. Capitol St, N.E., Rm 2224
Washington, DC 20002
202/442-9200

Florida Board of Pharmacy
John D. Taylor
Executive Director
4052 Bald Cypress Way, Bin #CO4
Tallahassee, FL 32399-3254
850/414-2969

Georgia State Board of Pharmacy
Anita O. Martin, Executive Director
237 Coliseum Drive
Macon, GA 31217-3858
478/207-1686

Guam Board of Examiners for Pharmacy
Teresita Villagomez, Acting Administrator
P.O. Box 2816
Hagatna, GU 96932
671/475-0251

Hawaii State Board of Pharmacy
Lee Ann Teshima, Executive Officer
P.O. Box 3469
Honolulu, HI 96801
808/586-2698

Idaho Board of Pharmacy
Richard "Mick" Markuson, Executive Director
PO Box 83720
Boise, ID 83720-0067
208/334-2356

Illinois Department of Professional Regulation
Sandra Dunn, Pharmacy Coordinator
320 W. Washington Street, 3rd Fl.
Springfield, IL 62786
217/785-8159

Indiana Board of Pharmacy
Kristen Burch, Director
402 W. Washington Street, Room 041
Indianapolis, IN 46204-2739
317/232-1140

Iowa Board of Pharmacy Examiners
Lloyd K. Jessen
Executive Secretary/Director
1209 E.Court, Executive Hills W.
Des Moines, IA 50319-0187
515/281-5944

Kansas State Board of Pharmacy
Carly Haynes, Acting Executive Director
Landon State Office Building
900 Jackson, Room 513
Topeka, KS 66612
785/296-4056

Kentucky Board of Pharmacy
Michael A. Moné, Executive Director
23 Millcreek Park
Frankfort, KY 40601-8204
502/573-1580

Louisiana Board of Pharmacy
Malcolm J. Broussard
Executive Director
5615 Corporate Blvd., Suite 8E,
Baton Rouge, LA 70808-2537
225/925-6496

Maine Board of Pharmacy
Geraldine Betts
Board Administrator
35 State House Station
Augusta, ME 04333
207/624-8603

Maryland Board of Pharmacy
LaVerne George Nasea, Executive Director
4201 Patterson Avenue
Baltimore, MD 21215-2299
410/764-4755

Massachusetts Board of Registration in Pharmacy
Charles R. Young
Executive Director
239 Causeway Street
Boston, MA 02113
617/727-9953

Michigan Board of Pharmacy
Cathy Seyka
Licensing Manager
611 W. Ottawa, 1st Fl.
P.O. Box 30670
Lansing, MI 48909-8170
517/373-9102

Minnesota Board of Pharmacy
David E. Holmstrom
Executive Director
2829 University Avenue S.E., Suite 530
Minneapolis, MN 55414-3251
612/617-2201

Mississippi State Board of Pharmacy
William L. Stevens
Executive Director
P.O. Box 24507
Jackson, MS 39225-4507
601/354-6750

Missouri Board of Pharmacy
Kevin E. Kinkade
Executive Director
P.O. Box 625
Jefferson City, MO 65102
573/751-0091

Montana Board of Pharmacy
Rebecca Deschamps, RPh, Executive Director
P.O. Box 200513
111 N. Jackson
Helena, MT 59620-0513
406/841-2356

Nebraska Board of Examiners in Pharmacy
Becky Wisell, Executive Secretary
P.O. Box 94986
Lincoln, NE 68509
402/471-2115

Nevada Board of Pharmacy
Keith W. Macdonald
Executive Secretary
555 Double Eagle Court
Suite 1100 Reno, NV 89511-8991
775/850-1440

New Hampshire Board of Pharmacy
Paul G. Boisseau
Executive Secretary
57 Regional Drive, Concord, NH 03301-8518
603/271-2350

New Jersey State Board of Pharmacy
H. Lee Gladstein
Executive Director
P.O. Box 45013
Newark, NJ 07101
973/504-6450

New Mexico Pharmacy Board
Jerry Montoya, Chief Inspector/Director
1650 University Blvd. N.E.
Suite 400B
Albuquerque, NM 87102
505/841-9102

New York Board of Pharmacy
Lawrence Mokhiber, Exec. Secy.
89 Washington Avenue, 2nd Floor West
Albany, NY 12234-1000
518/474-3817 ext. 130

North Carolina Board of Pharmacy
David R. Work
Executive Director
P.O. Box 459
Carrboro, NC 27510-0459
919/942-4454

North Dakota State Board of Pharmacy
Howard C. Anderson, Jr.
Executive Director
P.O. Box 1354
Bismarck, ND 58502-1354
701/328-9535

Ohio State Board of Pharmacy
William T. Winsley
Executive Director
77 S. High Street, Room 1702
Columbus, OH 43266
614/466-4143

Oklahoma State Board of Pharmacy
Bryan H. Potter
Executive Director
4545 Lincoln Blvd., Suite 112
Oklahoma City, OK 73105-3488
405/521-3815

Oregon State Board of Pharmacy
Gary A. Schnabel
Acting Executive Director
800 N.E. Oregon Street
#9 State Office Bldg., Room 425
Portland, OR 97232
503/731-4032

Pennsylvania State Board of Pharmacy
Melanie Zimmerman, Executive Secretary
124 Pine Street
P.O. Box 2649
Harrisburg, PA 17105-2649
717/783-7156

Puerto Rico Board of Pharmacy
Beverly Davila Morales
Executive Director
800 Avenida Robert T. Todd, Office #201, Stop 18
Santurce, PR 00908
787/725-8161

Rhode Island Board of Pharmacy
Richard A. Yacino
Chief3 Capitol Hill, Room 205
Providence, RI 02908
401/222-2837

South Carolina Board of Pharmacy
Cheryl A. Ruff, Administrator
P.O. Box 11927
Columbia, SC 29211-1927
803/896-4700

South Dakota State Board of Pharmacy
Dennis M. Jones
Executive Secretary
4305 S. Louise Ave., Suite 104
Sioux Falls, SD 57106
605/362-2738

Tennessee Board of Pharmacy
Kendall M. Lynch, Director
Second Floor
Davy Crockett Tower
500 James Robertson Parkway
Nashville, TN 37243
615/741-2718

Texas State Board of Pharmacy
Gay Dodson, Exec. Dir./Secy.
333 Guadalupe, Tower 3
Suite 600, Box 21
Austin, TX 78701-3942
512/305-8000

Utah Board of Pharmacy
A. Gary Bowen, Bureau Director
160 E. 300 South, P.O. Box 146741
Salt Lake City, UT 84114-6741
801/530-6767

Vermont Board of Pharmacy
Carla Preston, Staff Secretary
26 Terrace Street, Drawer 09
Montpelier, VT 05609-1106
802/828-2875

Virginia Board of Pharmacy
Elizabeth Scott Russell
Executive Director
6606 W. Broad Street, Suite 400
Richmond, VA 23230-1717
804/662-9911

Virgin Islands Board of Pharmacy
Lucien A. Moolenaar, Commissioner of Health
Roy L. Schneider Hospital, 48 Sugar Estate,
St. Thomas, VI 00802
340/774-0117

Washington State Board of Pharmacy
Donald H. Williams
Executive Director
P.O. Box 47863
Olympia, WA 98504-7863
360/236-4825

West Virginia Board of Pharmacy
William T. Douglass, Jr., Executive Director
232 Capitol Street
Charleston, WV 25301
304/558-0558

Wisconsin Pharmacy Examining Board
Patrick D. Braatz, Director
1400 E. Washington, P.O. Box 8935
Madison, WI 53708
608/266-2812

Wyoming State Board of Pharmacy
James T. Carder
Executive Director
1720 S. Poplar Street, Suite 4
Casper, WY 82601
307/234-0294